"*The 30-Day Faith Detox* is an awesome book. Not only does it talk about your body, which most detox books do, but it also talks about your soul and your spirit. Remember that your body was made in the image of God, and He wants you to care for it. This wonderful book will help you obtain wholeness in 30 days."

Dr. Marilyn Hickey, president, Marilyn Hickey Ministries

"We live in a world that is unpredictable. Life is real, and we all experience its ups and downs. Sometimes there are things that happen that can make us feel like we took two steps backward. But you never know what is just around the corner! In *The 30-Day Faith Detox*, Laura has provided the tools for us to apply disciplines in our everyday lives that will help us to be able to live freely and promote health in our body, soul and spirit."

Pastor Beni Johnson, Bethel Church, Redding, California;
author, *The Happy Intercessor* and *Healthy and Free*

"Excellent read—well written, relevant, compassionate and empowering for anyone looking for physical, mental, emotional and/or spiritual renewal. This should be a very important contribution in helping a large audience looking for a detox from life's many dietary, environmental and spiritual challenges."

Dr. Jim Sharps, N.D., H.D., Dr.N.Sc., Ph.D.; president
and CEO, International Institute of Original Medicine

"What we love most about Laura Harris Smith is that she passionately practices what she preaches (and writes!). She is a living model that *The 30-Day Faith Detox* actually works and will result in one's mind being renewed, body cleansed and spirit healed. As senior pastors, we are eager to challenge our church family to embark upon this 30-day detox and experience afresh the wholeness Jesus paid for us to enjoy. Laura's encouraging, easy-to-read instructions and insights

D0017522

make this journey delightful and doable. We heartily endorse *The 30-Day Faith Detox*."

Happy and Dianne Lehman, senior pastors, The Vineyard Church of Central Illinois; VUSA Executive Team members

"Laura Harris Smith is one of the most talented, creative, fun and interesting people I have ever met. I am amazed by how she continues to prove that over and over. With smoothie recipes like 'Brain Boosting Banana Choco Chip Smoothie' and 'The Bright Skin Blend,' Laura is now sure to become the Smoothie Queen!"

Paul McCulloch, franchise owner, Smoothie King International

"Hooked from the table of contents! I've read health-related detoxing books and materials for years, and I've known Laura through her health trauma and her intense faith. I pray this will be a bestseller. We all need it. This book is excellent! I began reading immediately and have already started my detox!"

Dr. Don Finto, founder and director emeritus, Caleb Company; pastor emeritus, Belmont Church, Nashville, Tennessee

"Laura Harris Smith has knocked it out of the park. This book is a spirit-, soul- and body-aligner. I love its simplicity yet great depth. You won't be disappointed."

Robby Dawkins, international conference speaker and evangelist; author, *Do What Jesus Did* and *Identity Thief*

THE 30-DAY FAITH DETOX

THE 30-DAY FAITH DETOX

RENEW YOUR MIND, CLEANSE YOUR BODY, HEAL YOUR SPIRIT

LAURA HARRIS SMITH

Chosen

a division of Baker Publishing Group
Minneapolis, Minnesota

© 2016 by Laura Harris Smith

Published by Chosen Books
11400 Hampshire Avenue South
Bloomington, Minnesota 55438
www.chosenbooks.com

Chosen Books is a division of
Baker Publishing Group, Grand Rapids, Michigan

Printed in the United States of America

ISBN 978-0-8007-9787-4 (pbk.)

Library of Congress Control Number: 2015952328.

The information given in The 30-Day Faith Detox is biblical, pastoral and spiritual in nature. It is not professional counsel and should not be viewed as such. Laura Harris Smith, Chosen Books and Baker Publishing Group specifically disclaim all responsibility for any liability, loss or risk, personal or otherwise, that is incurred as a consequence, directly or indirectly, of the use of and/or application of any contents of this book.

Cover design by Gearbox

16 17 18 19 20 21 22   8 7 6 5 4 3

To my father, Arlen, who taught me to eat color-
fully and to age with a healthy body.

To my mother, Adair, who taught me that a
decluttered house is a decluttered mind.

And to my husband, Chris, who attentively and
tenderly guards and cherishes my spirit.

If only everyone could have the three of you in their
lives this world would be a better place . . .
body, mind and spirit.

Contents

Use this private link for accessing free daily videos and weekly encouraging emails during your detox:

http://www.lauraharrissmith.com/faithdetox.html

Read Sections 1 and 2 first, and then go to that link when you are beginning Section 3, which is the actual first day of your detox. On that day, sign up for the free section emails, and they will come to you just as you are starting each new section. Also find your daily videos on that same web page.

Get access to daily support, testimonials and food preparation ideas, and meet faith detoxers from around the world, by joining the free Facebook group for *The 30-Day Faith Detox*:

https://www.facebook.com/groups/30DayFaithDetox

Faith and Physics

Faith can be fickle. If it were not for the fact that it is a spiritual gift from God, you might be tempted to think your faith has a mind of its own. One minute it is your biggest supporter, and the next minute it acts as if it does not even know your name. One day you have rallied enough faith to leap off mountains and breathe underwater, and the next day you cannot seem to force one foot in front of the other. And in that moment when it betrays you to the point that you are ready to betray God and abandon the very mission your faith dared you to embark upon, you find yourself having to confront that vanishing faith and say, "Get back here! You got me into this mess and you are going to get me out!"

But real faith does not make messes; it makes miracles. It is the currency of heaven and the means by which you purchase change for your life. Yes, Jesus paid it all, but Jesus cannot force you to want change. He cannot force you to have faith. He can order the circumstances of your life to cause you to need Him more, which sometimes leads to brushes with hopeless situations. But faith is the way of escape. Faith is Hope all dressed up with somewhere to go. It is Courage's child and Patience's twin.

You and I are here to discuss the current condition of your faith. It is the product of the previous troubles in your life and your response to each one. After each trial you decided either to get up and keep going, or to lie down, lower your expectations and alter your belief system. Each troubling challenge, with which life is teeming, left its residue upon your faith—good or bad—and affected your posture toward the ones to come. This book is about assessing the current condition of your faith and being honest about it with yourself and God to ensure that your faith is in optimal health and ready to greet the greatness He has for you.

Truth is, if you wrote a list of all the things that make you a great person of faith and another list of all your troubles, they would be the same list! Trouble hates faith because it does not get to be center stage anymore. But in between that time when trouble upstages your faith and your faith takes back the spotlight, that is where the real you steps forward. Faith lets you be you and God be God.

The Force of Faith

It has been said by many that faith stiffens you; that it is a mental starch that instantaneously prepares you to face any trial with great resolve. And if you are a believer in Jesus, that stiffening will become part of your everyday life. Faith is a fear stopper, and it will not let you let it die. Faith will nag and filibuster until you let it live again and conquer the trial before you. Faith is a stubborn force.

The title of this section is "Faith and Physics." What do physics and faith have in common? Physics is the science of three specific components: matter, energy and the interaction between them. Likewise, faith is the science of three components: spirit, mind and body. The way these three components relate is the foundation for this book. We will address how your spirit, mind and body affect your faith, and how to purge and position all three, resulting in a more forceful faith.

Physics requires matter and motion, but Scripture says that faith does, too. "Faith by itself, if it is not accompanied by action, is dead" (James 2:17 NIV), and "be ye doers of the word, and not hearers only" (James 1:22 KJV). So faith requires motion. Perhaps James was a physicist.

Count On It

If thinking scientifically about invisible faith is a stretch for you, then let's come up with a tangible equation for faith that you can see.

Algebra is the mathematical art of working with variables. In algebraic equations, letters represent variables; those letters are actually just numbers in disguise. We call them *variables* for an obvious reason: The numbers they represent may vary.

Even though I did rather well in algebra in high school, I did not enjoy it. So it pains me to tell you that life is just like algebra. (Yes, faith is like physics, and now life is like algebra.) As with algebra, there are countless problems in life that need solutions. We call them *variables* because they vary. Life comes with countless variables that can lead to unpredictable fluctuations in our faith. The terms of life, in fact, are the same as the terms used in algebra: irrational vs. rational, absolute values, intersections, deductive reasoning, common denominators and solutions. I suppose the only difference between algebra and life is that algebra has "constants"—and you do not need me to tell you that there is nothing constant about life except the Giver of it.

If faith is like physics and life is like algebra, then we can come up with an algebraic equation that makes faith tangible:

$$GP - D(H) + \frac{OC}{T} = PF$$

Can you decipher that? Look at it again carefully. It means "God's Promises minus Doubt multiplied by Hope plus Optimistic Confessions over Time equals Promises Fulfilled." Aaaaand . . . somebody out there just fell in love with algebra for the first time. Maybe physics, too.

Just as you have to learn to "speak" algebra or physics, so you have to learn to "speak" life. And to speak life, you have to learn faith. Faith—in its many expressions—is the alphabet of the language of life. By faith you can build words, and the words of that language will build your life. (And if you prefer language arts over science and math like me, this should be very good news to you.)

For All Intents and Purposes

The purpose of the next thirty days is to feed your faith, and to do that, we have to put your doubt on a diet. We have to put your flesh on a fast. You must decrease so He can increase. We are going to nourish your faith so that it can thrive, and starve your doubts so that they will die. Thirty days from now, your faith is going to be leaner, meaner and more intimidating to your enemy.

The purpose of the first two sections—Sections 1 and 2—is to prepare you for the thirty days themselves. They should be read a few days before beginning Section 3 so you can gather your supplies and prepare. These opening pages will prepare your mind, spirit, body, kitchen, faith, schedule and more. All put together, you will achieve a total "temple" cleansing, which will result in a stronger, purer you.

If you are facing the impossible right now in your life, or even just the mundane, you must fully grab hold of faith if you want change. Doubts are splinters in the fingers of your faith; they prevent you from taking a firm grip. My intent is for us to confront thirty common life adversities or setbacks that might, like splinters, interfere with your faith-grip. Thirty familiar trials you might have faced over the course of your lifetime that have put chinks in your faith, some from so long ago that you cannot even remember how they got there. You are going to step back and listen to your faith. It will be honest and tell you what condition it is in.

Why do you need faith? For two important reasons: God's pleasure and your possibilities: "Now without faith it is impossible to please God" (Hebrews 11:6 HCSB); "All things are possible for the one who has faith" (Mark 9:23 CEB). You see, God knows you want to have faith. It is what made you a Christian in the first place. So then why—if you already had faith in Jesus that resolved your impossible-to-fix eternal separation from God—do you sometimes struggle to believe that the impossible is possible in your everyday life?

When you feel the urge to have faith, it means that you are on God's mind right at that moment. It means He has a gift or opportunity for you that you must take His hand to go get. It means He believes in you. So faith is not a feeling. It is an offer. A tailor-made proposition. And faith only fails when you fail to have faith.

Nobody wants to live with doubt or fear, yet many Christians do. Nobody wants to be depressed or anxious, yet many Christians are. In our fallen world, the invisible toxins of doubt, disappointment, discouragement—plus the accumulation of what feels like unanswered prayer—can contaminate even the strongest faith, leaving behind symptoms that affect the spirit, mind and body, and leaving *the* Body of Jesus weakened and vulnerable.

Spirit, Mind and Body: Topics and Toxins

The thirty days of faith detoxification are divided into five categories, each receiving six days of focus. The categories are: (1) Social Influence Toxins, (2) Financial Toxins, (3) Health-Related Toxins, (4) Relationship Toxins and (5) Purpose and Identity Toxins.

Why five categories? Because in my near-thirty years of ministry I have found that anytime someone comes forward for prayer, the need falls into one of these five areas: prayers for social concerns, finances, health issues, relationships or a personal identity crisis. In one month's time, then, we will explore thirty universal faith-toxins that can infect you in spirit, mind and body, leaving you struggling.

How will each day look? First, with topics such as "When Healing Will Not Come," "Can't Seem to Get Ahead," "Fatal Faith (Losing Loved Ones)," "When Marriage Fails" and even "Catastrophic World Events," you will face your doubts head on, experience spiritual purging by embracing a biblical perspective on the issue, receive encouragement to keep standing (or to get back up) and learn Scriptures to use in prayer for change and progress.

Next, after each day's spiritual rehabilitation, the emotional pollutants will be addressed. The residues of fear, hopelessness, unforgiveness and more will be unmasked. Prayers and faith-filled declarations are included to bathe your mind and prepare it to sustain lasting change and growth. Emotional healing will follow.

Then, building upon the spiritual and emotional cleansing that has just occurred, we address the symptoms that oftentimes manifest physically as a result of the spiritual and emotional toxins. By following easy recipes of corresponding nutritional cleanses and using food as medicine, you will achieve a total body detox by the end of the month. Through the intake of liquid cleanses, smoothies, soups, hearty salads and detoxifying teas, your body will be healed of the toxic physical manifestations triggered by the correlating spiritual or emotional stress.

As we dig into each of the five categories noted above, we will cleanse three corresponding body organ systems. By the end of the thirty days, all fifteen of your major body systems will have been detoxed. Prayer by prayer, thought by thought and organ by organ, total cleansing comes to the whole temple, spirit, mind and body. First Corinthians 3:16 says, "Do you not know that you are God's temple and that God's Spirit dwells in you?"

Body Systems Detoxed

We will spend two days each on your fifteen body systems, gently cleansing them using organ-specific vegetables, fruits, liquids and nutrients. Here is the order in which we will cleanse.

- Digestive (mouth, esophagus, stomach, liver, large intestines)
- Excretory (small intestines, colon, rectum)
- Urinary (kidneys, bladder, gallbladder)
- Respiratory (nose, lungs, pharynx, larynx, trachea, bronchi, alveoli)
- Immune (bone marrow, thymus, glands)
- Lymphatic (spleen, lymph nodes, ducts, tonsils)
- Endocrine (hypothalamus, pituitary, thyroid, adrenals, pineal body)
- Nervous (brain, spinal cord, nerves)
- Reproductive (ovaries, testes)
- Cardiovascular (heart, blood vessels: arteries, capillaries, veins)
- Circulatory (blood, all vessels)

- Integumentary (skin, hair, nails, sweat glands)
- Skeletal (bones, bone marrow, joints, teeth, ligaments, cartilage)
- Muscular (muscles)
- Sensory (sight, hearing, feeling, smelling, tasting and balance)

Exercise

As we detox these fifteen body systems, please continue to exercise because it activates the entire lymphatic system, which in turn helps drain the toxins being removed from all the other body systems. It is probably not the time to start a vigorous new routine if you are decreasing your caloric intake, but definitely get moving! Twenty to thirty minutes a day of biking, walking or even time on an elliptical stepper or treadmill will serve you well.

Also, on some cable TV providers you can find free fitness workouts with every level of activity imaginable, from belly dancing to kickboxing and everything in between. Do not wait till Day 3. Get going and set new exercise habits that will stay with you long after the detox is completed! *But* remember to eat more if you move more this month.

Weighing In

Do not forget to weigh yourself at the beginning of the detox. Unless you have serious hormonal imbalances that prevent weight loss, you will see those numbers on the scales drop.

Now let's move on and discuss how we are going to accomplish this. Because the physical detoxification might be the most challenging component of our thirty days together, I want to spend a few minutes focusing on its importance, as well as reminding you of your body's intricate connection with your spirit and soul.

Cleaning House

This would be a good time to acknowledge that God has created several of your key organs to do all your detoxing for you. The liver, kidneys, skin and lungs are already excellent filters, for instance, capable of handling the typical environmental contaminants that throw themselves at your body (or hide in your food). Filters, however, get dirty. Overtaxed. So the purpose of the physical portion of this detox is to baby your body, disinfect your filtration system and free up your organs to do their jobs better.

Perhaps you have been to a doctor or nutritionist who has told you to lose weight. Perhaps you are getting ready for a photo shoot, a red carpet debut or trying to fit into that wedding attire. Maybe you have a high school reunion coming up that you want to look great for or a beauty pageant gown to fit into (been there, done that). Maybe you are an athlete with a nearing sports competition and you need that extra edge of lean, mean muscle. Whatever your reasons, this total body detox is for you.

Cleanses and detoxes reset the organs through tailor-made fasting. Yep, what you are about to embark upon can be considered a fast, even though it will not be an absolute fast (water only). I hope this might even redefine fasting for you.

If, however, at any time in the next thirty days you feel the need to go to the next level and eliminate solid foods for a few days, you can stick to the smoothies and/or juicing recipes, providing your doctor or nutritionist has no objections. Aside from the spiritual benefits, liquid fasting is a tremendous re-start button for your body. During fasting, the body rests and then uses recovered energy to begin repairing itself. Because of this, fasting is the most natural way—not to mention the speediest—to reverse disease, except, of course, if the body's cellular integrity has been irreversibly compromised. But even then, disease can be arrested and prevented from advancing.

Over the next thirty days you are going to refuel each organ with healthy nutrients that act like claws, literally digging out toxins and eliminating them from your body. This process will promote weight loss and advance elimination through the intestines, kidneys and skin, prompting your liver to expel toxins from your entire body. Fast! Have you lost your cheekbones and hipbones? Let's go find them!

There are some people who will buy this book solely for the thirty days of total body cleansing. The cleanses are non-intimidating and mentally stimulating. Ever perused those cookbooks that define "easy recipes" as "Lamb Haggis with Tarragon Turnips and Flambéed Aubergines"? Forget it! The mere title makes me want to shut the book and quit. I give you my word you will be able to pronounce everything in these recipes and find what you need at your local grocer.

I do encourage you to buy organic. Why? Think of it: It is no secret now that produce is typically sprayed with pesticides to keep the critters out and yield a better return. So what good does it do to detoxify your body while adding more toxins back in? Buy organic as often as possible. It seems more expensive until you count the money spent on doctor visits, medicine, home cures and work missed due to illnesses caused by eating poorly over time. Eat organic, eat local or grow it yourself. Your belly, budget and boss will thank you.

Every evening, if you feel you absolutely must, you have the option of eating three ounces of organic poultry or fish as long as it is free from all breading and bad oils. (I advocate the use of only olive, coconut, flaxseed or grapeseed oil for this detox program.) But you will be eating or drinking six times a day and will not be hungry, so do not give another thought to starvation.

According to a recent interview with Dr. Woodson Merrell on the *Dr. Oz Show*, the U.S. Centers for Disease Control reports that we each have approximately 140 toxic chemicals residing in us, and that these toxins are implicated in 70 percent of all chronic illness.[1] So, detoxing is beneficial.

Living Foods vs. Dead Foods

My father was a farmer, as was his father before him. From the time I was a little girl I have always remembered his having a garden, and I learned to eat every vegetable there was—a full rainbow variety of every color God puts into our fruits and vegetables. Daddy would come in from his garden with some new breed I had never heard of and say, "Baby, try it once and if you don't like it, you don't ever have to eat it again." So I would try. And I would like. Now, I eat the rainbow.

But years came, when I had small children of my own, when I opted for processed foods. They were quicker, easier and cheaper. They were the "dead foods" that sit in boxes, bags or cans in the middle of your grocery store, as opposed to living foods that line the walls and have to be refrigerated, such as produce, meats and dairy. If we would all shop along the periphery of our stores where the plug sockets are, we would be healthier.

Mark my words . . . processed foods are the new smoking. One day we will look back and wonder why we ever consumed them.

Not only did I begin eating a lot of processed foods, but I began working harder and demanding more from my body, including giving birth to six children. Plus, as I shared in my book, *Seeing the Voice of God: What God Is Telling You Through Dreams and Visions* (Chosen, 2014), I fell into an inherited habit of getting only four or five hours sleep a night. I accumulated a sleep debt that landed me on the brink of adrenal failure. And guess what? I *was* eating vegetables *and* exercising *and* avoiding bad fats. But I sort of dabbled at good health. It was not a daily priority anymore.

Sadly I think this describes most people. And we somehow expect our few good choices to outweigh all our bad ones. But that is like sewing a quilt with ripped fabric and not foreseeing the unraveling. And quilts do not have to undergo a fraction of the demands we put on our physical bodies in a single day. We are fearfully and wonderfully made. We should be fearfully and wonderfully taking care of ourselves.

Dying to Live

So there I was, in stage 3 adrenal burnout, and stage 4 is where all your organs shut down. Most of my body systems were already going awry. I had always been the picture of health. Slim, trim, vibrant, energetic. I was told regularly that I looked ten or fifteen years younger than I was. Now I felt old, haggard and in need of answers, fast. Whereas some people prefer blood tests, and others, saliva or urine tests, I got all three. And while some people prefer holistic nutritionists and others conventional doctors, I employed both. Call me a skeptic. Call me desperate.

Well, blood tests revealed my levels of TSH (thyroid stimulating hormone) were well into the hypothyroid range, confirmed by my body temperatures, which dipped down as low as 94.47 at times (normal being 98.6). This meant a sluggish metabolism, which eventually came to a screeching halt and resulted in weight gain. My reproductive system went crazy in my mid-thirties right after the birth of our sixth child. By my early forties it had shut down entirely. This led quickly to bone loss and two chipped teeth (after a lifetime with no cavities) and a broken rib in a freak accident.

My adrenals had all but quit producing cortisol (necessary to reduce stress) and adrenaline (necessary for energy). My digestive tract was not in great shape either, showing the presence of bad bacteria in my small intestines. My pancreas was throwing a temper tantrum, and my blood sugar, which had always been categorized as hypo-glycemic or low, suddenly pushed upward. Blood tests now revealed I was pre-diabetic. A multidecade battle with neurological misfiring in the form of small seizures, which had gotten better and better, had a sudden setback. Now I was having MRIs to test for pituitary tumors and hypothalamus malfunctions.

Most urgent of all, my liver and gallbladder appeared stressed. I was told they needed detoxing quickly, for with those filters clogged, my body could not benefit from the medicinal or supplemental regimens I needed for all of those other ailing body systems! I had a strange brain fog, my eyesight was failing, my skin was thinning and my hair was falling out. My calcium, vitamin D and antioxidant levels were dangerously low, and my morale and creative energy were plummeting right along with it.

My body's pH levels were very acidic (*pH* stands for "the power of hydrogen"), which could have been an indicator of all sorts of things, including kidney stones. And my kidneys definitely seemed stressed, based on a high specific gravity test that revealed abnormal leukocytes in my urine. The pH scale runs from 0 to 14, with a perfect balance being a neutral 7. Dipping below 7 indicates an acidic body and rising above 7 indicates an alkaline body. Most illnesses have a hard time thriving in a more alkaline body, while all sorts of illnesses are said to thrive in acidic bodies, including cancers. Some research indicates that the pH inside a tumor can be as low as 6. My pH registered down into the 5s, so I was definitely acidic, and at risk.

Multiple targeted stress tests showed that my body would not even stay in an alkalinized (safer) condition. In other words, my physical body was in what health professionals call a "hyper-vigilant state," which is an unending state of trying to fix itself. Healing was always just out of reach for my stressed body (not to mention my mind). Both were constantly busy. Imagine now the added danger from sleep deprivation. An immune system needs you to rest to be able to focus its entire attention on healing your body, and if you are busy all day and most of the night, too, your body will never, ever, *ever* heal properly. Sleep is the immune system's best friend.

Inflammation

What is inflammation? First of all, it is both good and bad; a necessary nuisance. Sort of like a headache is a nuisance, but its inflammation is necessary because it is a symptom that something is wrong elsewhere (even with migraines). Thereby, the headache becomes a clue—a gift—that sends us on the hunt to uncover the root reason for the inflammation, unless we just keep popping anti-inflammatories like ibuprofen (or any other pain killers) to mask the pain.

So that is the blessing and bother of inflammation, and my body was full of it, but if you need a more scientific definition, here it is: *Inflammation is the body's effort at self-protection.* Its goal is to rush healing to the scene of infirmity or injury and begin removing harmful irritants, stimuli and even unhealthy, damaged cells. It is our body's immune system in action. Whenever harm or sickness comes, inside or out, inflammation is the biological reaction to remove that harm and begin the process of repair. My entire body was full of inflammation, working desperately toward healing.

You might have thought of inflammation as the sore, swollen redness that follows stubbing your toe, which it is, but more. True, when you stub your toe it becomes red, sore and perhaps swollen, but that is because your immune system is rushing blood to the scene of the injury in an attempt to mend it. The soreness has a source and the redness has a reason. Healing is on the way!

But now imagine that an injury or infirmity has occurred on the inside of your body. Maybe the "stubbed toe" is in one of your internal organs through the form of illness or an internal injury. Though unseen, it is still present, and your divinely discerning immune system will not rest until it sees healing come.

The trouble with chronic illnesses is that the body lives in a constant state of inflammation, which makes the immune system work overtime; thus, it is in a constant state of reaction. This can actually be measured by a blood test called the C-reactive protein test (CRP). Most often administered to determine the risk of heart disease or stroke, it can also be used to measure inflammation since this special protein increases in the bloodstream when any type of bodily inflammation is present. A very low pH, which I had, is also a measure of acute inflammation.

If you are interested in testing your own pH levels, you can buy pHydrion strips at most drugstores (or order them online) and test your urine and saliva, comparing the color change on the strip to the enclosed results chart. Waking urine and saliva are best since the body is more acidic the earlier your measure, and you want to get a snapshot of what your most acidic (and dangerous) levels are. Totally neutral is a level of 7 in both, with ideal urine readings being between 6.5–7.0 and ideal saliva results being between 7.0–7.5. And remember, the cure for acidic pH levels is to consume more vegetables and fruits, which you are about to do!

What I Took Out

With the help of skilled nutritionist (and degreed scientist) Anne Reed, M.S., N.C., I first addressed my diet. With my body working so hard to heal, I had to give it less to do digestively, which meant ridding my diet of hard-to-process foods. Namely, wheat. As of late 2012 I have removed all gluten from my diet. Of course, gluten is in just about everything (even some lip glosses), and so it is impossible to say I have had none at all. But it is no longer on the menu of my life. Why so extreme for someone who does not have celiac disease?

Basically gluten is the "glue" that makes bread doughy, and it is a mixture of two proteins found in certain grains, especially wheat. I remember thinking, *What is so bad about wheat? Jesus spoke well of wheat. He even compared Christians to it, right?* But the truth is, today's wheat ain't your grandma's wheat—and it certainly is not Jesus'. It is not the wheat from a thousand, a hundred or even sixty years ago.

In an effort to create massive amounts of wheat for lower costs and greater profits, modern grain processors have figured out a way to separate the nutritious components of grain (the germ and bran) from the endosperm where most of the carbs are found. This genetic modification has resulted in a marked reduction in nutrient density—not to mention the fact that today's refined bread can contain multiple times more gluten than former bread, a level our bodies were never designed by God to digest.

So they do not digest. Yes, sometimes the gluten in your breads and pastas just sits in your gut and rots. As a result, today's refined wheat breads are super-inflammatory.

This "refining" also causes today's wheat to make blood sugar levels spike very quickly. Such spikes wreak havoc on the body. Enormous internal energy has to be focused on calming down this reaction, even in the healthiest bodies. In my case, with my pancreas and liver already working overtime to heal their inflammation, giving them one more thing to do was like Pharaoh demanding the Hebrew slaves make more bricks out of less straw. So I gave my body a gift and gave up wheat. It has thanked me repeatedly ever since. Weight loss. More energy. And the obliteration of my bloat.

I also gave up sugar. My nutritionist told me it was vital. That makes sense because if wheat converts to sugar and causes sharp blood sugar spikes, it would not do any good to give up wheat and still eat sugar, which obviously causes sugar spikes!

What I Put Back In

There is practically no recipe or dish I had before that I cannot enjoy now; it just means substituting the wheat and sugar with simple ingredients of my choice. I enjoy the natural sweetness of stevia, honey, coconut crystals and natural xylitol, and I do not feel I am missing a single, solitary thing. I still eat bread, too, but in place of wheat flour I use almond, rice and other flours.

Now that I know what to buy, those items are on my beaten path at my local grocery store. And even though the bodily crisis is over and my immune system is not working overtime to stop inflammation, I have chosen not to go back to wheat and sugar. Why would I? I am not going back to Egypt.

I also began taking some wonderful supplements as I rebuilt my diet to once again eat the rainbow, as my father taught me to do. And most importantly, I changed my sleep health. I was actually put on strict bed rest at one point. In fact I wrote *Seeing the Voice of God* on total bed rest, so its success can only be attributed to the grace and goodness of God, trust me. I could feel the point at which my inflammation brain fog began to lift in my recovery. I knew I was writing that book in the middle of a miracle. I was right. And now I am humbled when I read online reviews from readers who say that miracles came to them too while reading it. The miracles are even finding their way into our ministry conferences. Only God can do that! He took my mess and turned it into a message!

Within six months my adrenals, no longer exhausted, were helping fuel the rest of my body toward healing. Within a little more than a year, a C-reactive protein test showed that there was no more inflammation left in my system! An added surprise was that a lifetime of seasonal and animal allergies vanished. Whereas cats and dogs used to send me to the ER with hives, breathing difficulties and more, now all four-footed creatures are my friends. For the first time in my life I can pet a cat, pat a dog and touch a live Christmas tree. This happened as a result of removing inflammatory foods from my diet, replacing them with better ones, and detoxing my system. Organ by organ, I detoxed my entire body. Day by day, week by week and month by month, I am now experiencing the healthiest years of my life as I enter my fifties.

Why I Can Help You

Spiritually: It is true that I am an ordained pastor, but you can call me a shepherdess like Rachel or Zipporah if it better agrees with your theology. I am not a "titles" person; it does not matter one bit to me as long as I get to keep herding sheep. Counting the time before and since my ordination as a sheepherder, I have spent the last 25 years of my life making myself available to people for spiritual support. If you count the fact that I was spiritually advising schoolmates in organized settings since junior high school, the figure jumps to more than 35 years. I have prayed with, fasted for, prophesied over and cried alongside daughters, sons, fathers, mothers, husbands and wives about their daughters, sons, fathers, mothers, husbands and wives.

I have seen sin patterns promptly halted, addictions broken, marriages mended, generational curses reversed, families restored, sad hearts encouraged, financial matters resolved, the Holy Spirit poured out and lives rebuilt.

I have seen miracles manifest before my very eyes. To God's glory I have laid my hands on people and had physical vision restored, deaf ears opened, cancers eradicated, HIV reversed, chronic pain disappear, barren wombs open, medical diagnoses reversed and much more. I have watched a leg grow by inches into my hands; I heard the bones popping from the spine to the hip as it happened. It is true. I have no reason to lie to you or try to impress you, and I have God to answer to if I attempt either.

It is my life's work, as thankless as it sometimes may be. My husband and I are bi-vocational pastors and individually receive small stipends from our church. We do what we do because God has "brainwashed" us to love and help people whether or not they love or help us back. Thank God, most do. They see our hearts. They know that we feel failure when they fail and feel like winners when they win. We love "doing life" with people. So I want you to feel that I am doing life with you while you are reading this book and following this faith detox. I am praying for you.

Emotionally: Because of the countless souls I have knelt with, I have learned how to counsel, confront and care for just about every personality type. I have learned to employ the spiritual gift of discernment of spirits quickly to expedite any session. I do not like mincing words. I disdain wasting time. I like seeing people changed, and I can tell in the first few minutes if they really want change. If they do not, I have been known to tell them to come back when they are ready. Not much happens until they are serious about change, so I had rather clear the time for someone who really is. Your purchasing this book shows you are.

Physically: As for helping you in your body, my second chance at life with better nutrition led to me back to school to become a C.N.C. (certified nutrition counselor). It was a natural extension of my new appreciation for biblical nutrition. That decision was not so I could become a practicing nutritionist, but rather to help educate you, my readers, on the importance of "original medicine."

If you had told me back when I was detoxing my organs and fighting for my life that I would one day become certified to use that same information to help others, I would not have believed you. I was too busy trying to live, learn, unlearn and pray for God's intervention so that my husband did not have to finish raising our children alone. I certainly could not have recognized that I was stockpiling culinary revelations that would one day help others. In fact, someone once prophesied over me that I would one day write a cookbook. Seeing as how I hate to cook, I literally laughed out loud. Now here I am. I cannot remember who that person was, but perhaps the first recipe here should have something to do with eating crow.

Here is what I know: Medicine did not heal me; food healed me. God's food. I had no prescriptions that brought me back from the brink of death. Not that conventional medicine is bad; I assure you I am *not* anti-medicine. Nor do I want you to be. But even if there had been prescriptions that could have cured my failing organ systems, my body still would have been depleted of the nutrients it needed—nutrients that would not have been found in those prescriptions. The result would have been an endless cycle of medicating new symptoms. Only the nutrients God made on the third day of creation and placed in plants, herbs, minerals, fruits and vitamins brought me total wholeness, which is broader than healing.

As I was praying for the supernatural to appear, God instead decided to add His super to my natural and let me participate in my recovery. He required me to cooperate with Him by discovering and partaking in the health He had placed in foods thousands of years before I ever needed them. That way I could maintain my miracle.

And I have.

Double-Check

First, I expect you to check with your doctor or nutritionist before beginning this detox. Especially if you

- are pregnant or nursing
- have active cancer
- have food allergies
- have a mental illness
- are under eighteen
- have liver disease or hepatitis
- have type 1 diabetes
- are on medications for bipolar disorder
- have an allergy to any food or ingredient listed here

If you have a medical condition, see your physician or nutritionist before starting this program.

This detox program is not intended, of course, to diagnose, treat, cure or prevent any disease. Tell your doctor that you will be using detoxifying foods to nourish your body for thirty days. I think he or she will be happy that you are improving your nutrition. If your doctor has any concerns about preexisting conditions, make sure to take those into consideration. Tell your doctor you will *not* be coming off any of your medications, and tell your nutritionist that you will remain on all of your supplements.

And check your medications carefully for interactions. Grapefruit, for instance, can sometimes interfere with cholesterol statin medications, as well as HIV medications, calcium channel blockers (blood pressure drugs), antihistamines, pain medications and psychiatric drugs. If you are on any of those (or other drugs) you probably already know which foods to avoid, but just double-check with your doctor. He or she is well versed in the Hippocratic oath and will know that it was Hippocrates himself who said, "Let food be thy medicine and medicine be thy food"!

The Gut-Brain Link

Did you know there is a link between your stomach and your thoughts? Have you ever had a "gut reaction" or a "gut feeling"? What about all those other idioms such as "hating someone's guts," "spilling your guts" or "going with your gut"? How about the simple feeling of having "a nervous stomach" or "butterflies in your stomach" or experiencing such severe anxiety with stage fright that you want to throw up? Do you think there is any link between your stomach and brain? Science says yes.

An article entitled "The Gut-Brain Connection" in a Harvard Medical School health publication explains the following:

> The brain has a direct effect on the stomach. For example, the very thought of eating can release the stomach's juices before food gets there. This connection goes both ways. A troubled intestine can send signals to the brain, just as a troubled brain can send signals to the gut. Therefore, a person's stomach or intestinal distress can be the cause *or* the product of anxiety, stress, or depression. That is because the brain and the gastro-intestinal (GI) system are intimately connected—so intimately that they should be viewed as one system.[2]

Did you catch that? "Intestinal distress can be the cause *or* the product of anxiety, stress, or depression." So if we could put an end to your intestinal distress, could we possibly eradicate your anxieties, stress symptoms and depressions? Could we at least improve them? Conversely, could we improve or even eradicate many GI conditions by reducing stress? Listen to the Harvard article's thoughts on the matter:

Based on these observations, you might expect that at least some patients with functional GI conditions might improve with therapy to reduce stress or treat anxiety or depression. And sure enough, a review of 13 studies showed that patients who tried psychologically based approaches had greater improvement in their digestive symptoms compared with patients who received conventional medical treatment.

If science is confirming the intimate link between stomach and brain, then surely what goes into the stomach (food and drink) can affect what goes on in the brain (thought and personality). This means that what you eat affects what you think and what you think affects what you eat. Simply put, your food impacts your thoughts.

The Food-Faith Link

So, then, consider this question: Is it possible that your thoughts can affect your faith? Because if so, then we can take it to the next step and make the case that your food affects your faith. Let me unpack that for you. Harvard has stated that "the brain and the gastrointestinal (GI) system are intimately connected—so intimately that they should be viewed as one system." This means that what happens in one affects the other. One processes food and one processes thoughts. Thus, it is easy to see how foods and thoughts can impact one another. So if it has been suggested that what you eat affects what you think, and if it can be proven biblically that what you think affects your faith, then it can be said that what you are eating is currently affecting your faith.

Think of it. You could—at this very moment—be chemically driving yourself toward doubt. Having a bad day? Thinking negative thoughts? Having a hard time mustering up a mustard seed? What if it is something you ate last night? Spiritual food poisoning.

This is not to minimize the influence of demonic interference with our faith. Sometimes we wrestle against evil spirits to maintain our faith on a daily basis. But remember, we are three parts—spirit, mind and body—and so we should not be surprised at how they are interdependent upon each other for total temple health.

So let's listen to what the Bible says about the connection between faith and thoughts. James 1:3–8 defines doubt as "double-mindedness," indicating that the mind can affect our faith: "But let him ask in faith, with no doubting, for the one who doubts is like a wave of the sea that is driven and tossed by the wind. For that person must not suppose that he will receive anything from the Lord" (James 1:6–7).

And Philippians 3:15 shows that maturing faith and thoughts are intertwined: "Whoever has a mature faith should think this way. And if you think differently, God will show you how to think" (GWT).

And finally, Isaiah 26:3 seems to link trust in God with thoughts: "You [God] keep him in perfect peace whose mind is stayed on you, because he trusts in you."

It is no surprise to me that science is proving "the brain and the gastrointestinal (GI) system are intimately connected—so intimately that they should be viewed as one system." Think of how fasting affects your faith as evidence of this. True fasting involves the removal of some or all foods from the diet—accompanied by prayer—and anytime I have ever fasted I have gone to a new place in my faith. Perhaps there is a physiological reason for this deepening of faith: Detoxing and cleansing the stomach results in clearer thinking and sharper faith. Again, that is not to undermine the spiritual miracle of fasting. It is just to confirm that the gut-brain link might also provide a food-faith link.

Look at these closing Scriptures in a new light and see if perhaps they link food with faith, or with doubt for that matter:

"Whoever has doubts is condemned if he eats, because the eating is not from faith. For whatever does not proceed from faith is sin" (Romans 14:23); "Man shall not live by bread alone, but by every word that proceeds from the mouth of God" (Matthew 4:4 NKJV).

So as you can see, the physical detoxes we will be undertaking are not just an addendum to the corresponding spiritual and emotional cleansing you will complete each of the thirty days. We are focusing on the physical aspect because what you eat could be affecting your thoughts and faith, and, thus, could be chemically propelling you toward doubt. If so, in thirty days, we are going to change the chemistry of your body and—along with spiritual and emotional cleansing—detox your faith!

When I sit with individuals pastorally at Eastgate Creative Christian Fellowship, where my husband and I minister in Nashville, Tennessee, I ask them the hard questions about spirit, mind and body. I help them set goals. In my decades of spiritually counseling others, I have seen marriages restored, peace reclaimed, children come home, depression end, weight lost, bodies healed, new careers birthed and much more. I want to do the same for you as if I am sitting with you and pastoring you.

Are you ready to get to work?

SECTION 2

Prepare to Be Amazed

In case you are wondering what we can really accomplish in your spirit, body and mind in thirty short days, let's start with an analogy.

What Can Thirty Days Really Do?

Suppose that as of today you make a choice. Let's say you are emotionally tired of holding out hope for a better life. You decide to throw caution to the wind, throw in the towel and throw away your goals for bettering yourself.

Then let's say you decide that forgiving others has gotten you nowhere in life, and so you drudge up every grudge you have ever felt and then feed them. You go back through the embarrassing memories of your school days, run-ins with former work associates, confrontations at family gatherings. You even recall disputes with pesky neighbors. You make a record of wrongs with those who have hurt you and revisit every offense. Then you decide to call each and every person and issue retribution. Many of them retaliate in defense, and new and even greater animosities arise. Bridges are burned.

Spiritually, you feel God's displeasure from the toxic unforgivenesses, so you express your anger at Him, too, and reject His voice. You remind Him of every prayer that did not get answered the way you wanted and of every penny you gave in the offering plate that did not seem to come with any return. There really is plenty of "fruit" from your prayers and your giving, but at this point, you cannot see it. You quit going to church because it is too convicting, delete all your social media friends who remind you of church or of God, quit reading your Bible, unsubscribe from all online Christian devotionals . . . and you hide. Bitterness is born.

Physically, your body begins to show the signs of this spiritual and emotional poisoning. The venom spreads rapidly to your health choices. You find yourself settling for the temporary happiness of comfort foods and partake of them often. Because of the lack of peace in your life, you now need a glass of wine each night to get to sleep, then eventually two or three. You slip into depression. This leads you to visit your doctor, who gives you medications to help you sleep, and, eventually, stimulants to help jumpstart your now slowing metabolism.

By the end of just one month, your face, ankles and midsection are swollen and distended from poor nutritional choices, and your weight has increased—not to mention the heaviness you feel because you have disfellowshipped God from your life. The burden of the other severed personal relationships is also like a millstone around your neck. The loss of friends who once brought you joy has taken you to a new low of grief and agony. You even have a passing thought of taking your life.

The Miracle Month

Wow! Do you see the changes you could make in yourself in just thirty days? Now turn that around and imagine the good you could do in that same amount of time!

You could get to the bottom of traumas and trials that have caused a lull in your faith. You could confront your doubts and figure out where they came from, putting them to rest forever as you reconcile them to God's Word. You could find peace with what you consider to be unanswered prayer, and see your hope revived. You could see those prayers answered forthrightly because of the new condition of your faith and trust in God's power.

You could also examine your personal relationships and see which are good for you and which are not. You could learn how to respond to people who try your patience and get on your last nerve. You could go deeper in forgiveness and watch God work out situations you cannot handle in your own strength. You could also learn to receive love in ways that would change your sense of self-worth forever.

But you will probably see the most immediate tangible results in your physical body as you flush out, rehydrate, liquidate and eliminate. Imagine it with me: sleeping better and going from exhausted to excited as you notice the results in the mirror. Expelling your swell, blasting your bulge, and going from frazzled to refreshed and from weary to *wow*. Picture yourself zapping your cellulite, sliding off your snug rings, and recovering a radiant complexion as you establish a healthier lifestyle.

For good this time.

This is big. You have an appointment with your future. You need to make a vow to devote the next thirty days to yourself and to God and not compromise them. Gentlemen, let me ask you: Would you opt for an evening with the guys to go eat hot wings rather than witness the birth of your first child? Ladies:

Would you go get ice cream instead of attending your parent's funeral? No, because you know how to set priorities. Right now, *you* are what is important. You can make the decision for one month not to go along with what others want to do or eat what they want to eat. Take back your body, mind and spiritual future. You have a job to do, and I am going to help you do it. Stat.

720 Hours: Three Challenges

Within these thirty days are 720 hours. Of those 720 hours you need to spend 270 of them sleeping. Yes, that is nine hours per night. You are saying, "No way!" To which I respond, "*Yes* way!" Doubt and unbelief take a significant toll on the body. Worry brings insomnia. Faith brings rest. So we are going to have to retrain your circadian rhythms over the next month and teach you to rest in true peace again. If you will adhere to this, you will still have 450 waking hours to concentrate on healing your body, your mind and your spirit.

And here is another challenge for you to get maximum benefit from this faith detox: Give God a tithe of your waking hours during this month. That is right, 10 percent of those 450 waking hours. In other words, aim to spend 45 hours on "God and you time." That is 1.5 hours per day. And you are going to need it.

Here is how you could break that down. Divide those ninety minutes into three thirty-minute increments. Spend the first thirty minutes reading that day's detox devotional text and planning the food detoxes for the day. Later in the same day, spend another thirty minutes in prayer asking God to show you any place where what you read has affected you spiritually. You will begin during this time to sense God working to heal your spirit. Then that evening, spend another thirty minutes praying about the emotional challenges from that day's devotional focus. Remember that your body will be detoxing all day long as you consume each cleansing food or drink.

Just imagine how this will affect your prayer life when you have completed these thirty days. You will have established a new habit of being able to sit with the Lord and wait on Him, listen and receive revelation from Him.

Are you ready to give Him a tithe of your waking hours? While the detoxes and cleanses will change your body, it is these 45 hours that will most bolster the good changes happening in your spirit and mind.

Now let's move on and discuss how we are going to accomplish this.

Prepare Your Kitchen

I am excited for you as you press toward your total temple transformation. While spiritual and emotional detoxing can be a private, internal process, the cleansing of your body will bring results that everyone can see, and they may come quicker than you would think.

We need to get your kitchen ready for this journey. You will be enjoying calming teas, friendly soups, cellulite-busting smoothies, colorful salads and scrumptious shakes.

Because of the multiple toxins, steroids and antibiotics that accumulate in the fatty tissues of animal flesh, meat consumption has become a risky business. Knowing that some of you will desire meat occasionally, I want to make sure you understand how to do this in the most healthy way possible so that you do not run the risk of putting more toxins back in (which is easy to do with today's meats) while you are working so hard to remove them with your vegetables. This would be the equivalent of trying to brush your teeth while eating Oreos! Just decide that you will select only organic meat that is humanely raised and fed. Remember: You are what you eat eats. If you will do this now, you will do it after the detox and never go back to dirty foods. Food is medicine. Before *and* after detoxing.

Making room: You will want to clean out your pantry to let go of the dead foods you always reach for when you're hungry and rushed. Trash those chips, cookies and other boxed foods. Also, purge your fridge to make space for the good foods you will be eating—and to lessen the temptation to deviate from your detox program. Go ahead and throw out those containers of fast-food leftovers, and surrender all those secret candy stashes hidden in drawers and cupboards. Come on! No excuses!

Water: No tap water during this time. Fridge filters rarely catch even a fraction of the harmful microbes and bacteria in water. Preferably, you will go one step further and invest in an under-the-counter water filtering system. Mine cost about $130, and I can feel my organs thanking me each day. This one small commitment gave my filtering organs less to filter so that they could concentrate on all the other unpredictable toxins out there.

At the very, very least, you could purchase purified water in jugs, although at the end of the month you will have paid for a good chunk of a new water system! You should drink half of your body weight in ounces each day. If you weigh 150 pounds that is 75 ounces. A sure sign that you are getting enough water on this detox is if you are using the bathroom once every hour or two.

Sweeteners: No sugar. Refined sugars are bad for multiple reasons. It can lead to diabetes, obesity and higher cholesterol. It can overload the liver with high fructose levels, lead to insulin resistance and cause constant elevated insulin levels, which contribute to cancer.

And did I mention that it is highly addictive? You do not need me to tell you that. But you might not know that sugar triggers a massive dopamine release in the brain. This pharmacological response can lead to serious (and yet socially acceptable) addiction. For some people, moderation will not do; they must practice total abstinence from sugar. For the next thirty days, that is you. And remember: Organic sugar is still sugar! Please avoid it.

Instead enjoy the following sweeteners on this detox: stevia in its many forms (powder, leaves, liquid), agave, honey, xylitol. Add them to any smoothie or liquid to give it a sweet boost. It only takes a little! (These are not measured equally to sugar.)

Spices: Feel free to mix in any herb or spice to the recipes any time. Cinnamon is an especially yummy addition to just about anything. Other flavor enhancers are chili powder, onion powder, cayenne powder, dill, cumin, ginger, basil, parsley, thyme and rosemary. Now is the time to go through your spice cabinet and replace your stale spices for optimum health benefits.

I know you will find the recipes to be delicious, but remember, they *are* your medicine. This is a detox! So doctor the recipes if you must, but your last result is to hold your nose and chug. Stick with the program.

Prepare Your Appliances

Here are some appliances you will need.

Blender: You will definitely need this for the smoothies. Blenders can be purchased very inexpensively (sometimes around $10 for a basic model).

Juicer: This would be beneficial due to the endless possibilities it provides for detoxifying drinks (a very low-end juicer can be purchased for around $20).

Teakettle: Or any electronic device that can boil water.

Stockpot: You are going to fix lots of soup, so you will want a small stockpot. Big enough to hold several servings but small enough that you can still stick it in the refrigerator and reheat.

And here is one appliance you will *not* need:

Microwave: You will not need a microwave in the next month. I hope that you will learn you can live without it! Reheat all soups and teas on the stovetop. Many scientific studies have stated the detrimental effects of microwaves on nutrition, urging that microwaves cause vegetables to lose antioxidants and vitamins, make healthful properties inert, "unfold" proteins and basically kill your food. Other studies disagree, stating that no harm is done whatsoever.

Microwaves do, however, produce radiation, which many believe can leak and cause harm. Since the opinions on this issue are so polarized and the stakes are so high, I decided to invest in an electromagnetic radiation meter to do my own microwave study. These meters are not cheap, and I wanted the best, so my daughter Jessica and I went in on one together. The FDA, which enforces strict microwave safety guidelines, states: "Most ovens tested show little or no detectable microwave leakage."[1] But my own two microwaves painted a drastically different picture, and so did Jessica's.

We tested one large counter model, one small counter model and one over-the-range model. The industry-trusted meter we purchased, when placed on the doors of all three microwaves while operating, registered so high that the meter arm was stuck to the right of the red-zone "HIGH" range, far beyond the last registrable measurements. In other words, the radiation was off the charts—well beyond what is generally recognized as safe.[2] To double-check my statistics of my own microwaves, I got a second, smaller meter—this one digital—and performed the same test. It also showed abnormally high levels of microwave leakage.

My personal hypothesis, therefore, is that the FDA has wishful thinking concerning microwave radiation leakage, but that in the end, more is emitted than we know. And if that is what is happening on the outside of the microwave, how can it be any healthier for the foods with living phytonutrients on the inside of it? The same FDA article also says, "It is known that microwave radiation can heat body tissue the same way it heats food." So, despite what side you are on in this heated debate (pun intended), I hope we all agree that you should not be standing in front of your microwave staring at your food as it cooks (if you use the microwave at all). In my test, the radiation levels were still in the dangerous red zone when I stepped four feet away from the microwave while it was cooking, and I could not get into a safe zone without leaving the kitchen entirely.

I encourage you to fall in love again with your stovetop and oven. Both will come in handy during this detox. I also purchased an inexpensive convection toaster oven a few years ago and love it!

Prepare and Compare Your Lists

I do not have to tell you to read labels carefully during this detox, because you are not going to be eating much of anything that comes with a label! You will be eating all living foods, or soups or drinks created from them. And you can eat those freely.

Here is a list of items to abstain from entirely during the next thirty days (at least), and a list of those to enjoy.

"No, Thanks" List

- Alcohol, sodas, nicotine
- Coffee, except for beans in smoothies
- Sugar and artificial sweeteners
- Wheat and gluten
- Cereals, any packaged foods
- Candies, chocolates
- Chips, crackers

- Fast food
- Canned food
- Margarine and "spreads"
- Beef and pork
- MSG
- Corn oil, canola oil, vegetable oils
- Cheese

"Yes, Please" List

- Vegetables, organic
- Fruits, organic
- Brown rice, quinoa (or any quinoa product, including quinoa pasta)
- Beans, lentils
- Green tea (decaf)
- Organic poultry or fish (although you are urged to do the detox "veggie-style")
- Olive, coconut, flaxseed, grapeseed oils
- Plain almond, organic 2%, rice and coconut milks
- Dried and fresh herbs and spices
- Apple cider vinegar
- Himalayan pink* and sea salt
- Butter (vegan or dairy)
- Filtered water (no tap)
- Stevia, agave, xylitol, local organic honey

*Preferred, as it contains more than 84 minerals and vitamins. Himalayan pink salt is like a multivitamin in your salt! Avoid iodized tablet salt because it is highly refined, heavily processed and contains anti-clumping agents.

The Veggie-Hater's Guide

But what if you simply hate vegetables (or fruits) or their by-products on your "Yes, please" list?

If you have always felt this way, you have been a victim of bad vegetables. Either badly grown, badly stored or badly prepared. Do you even know how many different types of fruits and vegetables there are? What if I told you there are some four thousand? Would that give you hope that surely there are a few you might like?

No? Then let me broaden the range! The number four thousand is merely the number of known tomato species. There are more than five thousand species of potatoes. And at one time there were more than seven thousand varieties of apples. So you see, there is no way to count the number of vegetables or fruits you could try, but the point is that *surely* there are some you can learn to enjoy.

The Vegetable/Fruit Challenge

So I have eight great challenges for you veggie-haters.

1. Stop saying you hate vegetables. The power of death is in your tongue (see Proverbs 18:21). Every time you proclaim this hatred, the enemy smiles and plots the order of the infirmities he hopes to layer into your life. Instead, pray the prayer included below for God to change your palate. Pray it daily until you see change, no matter how long it takes.

2. Former veggie-haters often describe finding a desirable "gateway vegetable" and then beginning to enjoy others in the same family. Find your gateway vegetable and start experimenting.

3. When eating out, try just one bite of something on a friend's plate each time. Eventually you will find things you like and can begin ordering them yourself.

4. Mask the taste and texture of vegetables by hiding them in other foods. You can Google endless recipes and tricks on how to do this.

5. Try the "fork load method." Serve veggies on your plate and put a small piece in with each forkful of something else.

6. Discover your oven's secret setting: Broil! Slice chips from a vegetable with a mandolin slicer and toss them in olive oil and sea or pink salt. Place in a thin layer under the broiler, watching closely so they do not burn. You will enjoy crisp veggies without the calories of frying. See "Tam's To-Your-Health Roasted Vegetables" in our recipe section for directions on roasting larger wedges of vegetables.

7. For the next four weeks, find one new vegetable each week that you will eat (not juice or blend, but eat).

8. Likewise, take the fruit challenge: For the next four weeks, find one new fruit to eat (not just juice or blend). When sliced and gently sautéed in olive oil or butter on medium high heat until golden brown, the sugar in fruit decomposes or "caramelizes." Pears, peaches, bananas, apples and more can be caramelized, but start with firm fruit because it does soften internally during the process.

When the above methods work for you, especially when you conquer the veggie and fruit challenges, please tell the world (and me) on my Facebook page (www.Facebook.com/Laura HarrisSmithPage)! Post pictures of yourself with your favorite new fruit and/or vegetables, whether it be a root or shoot. I cannot wait to hear from you! Share your recipes for casseroles, smoothies, juice-blends, soups, etc. I am going to see each one personally and smile!

Why It Matters

Now that I have encouraged you to explore the wonderful tastes and benefits of vegetables and fruit, I have to level with you and deliver some bad news. If you never eat vegetables, you will most likely die earlier than you are intended to. It is your choice because God has given you free will to choose, but here is what He intended for you: "And God said, 'Behold, I have given you every plant yielding seed that is on the face of all the earth, and every tree with seed in its fruit. You shall have them for food'" (Genesis 1:29).

When God says, "It shall be," whether He is creating the world, speaking light into the darkness or raising the dead, He *wants* it to be. He has a reason for it to be. In the case of vegetables and fruits, they alone contain God's medicines that make you immune to Satan's illnesses. Science backs this up: According to the *Journal of Epidemiology & Community Health*,

> Researchers used the Health Survey for England to study the eating habits of 65,226 people representative of the English population between 2001 and 2013, and found that the more fruit and vegetables they ate, the less likely they were to die at any age. Eating seven or more portions reduces the specific risks of death by cancer and heart disease by 25% and 31% respectively. The research also showed that vegetables have significantly higher health benefits than fruit.[3]

And I have some more bad news: Potatoes and corn are not nutritionally considered vegetables. Sorry. Potatoes are botanically classified as vegetables but nutritionally labeled as a starch (like pasta, rice or bread). Dried corn is considered a grain and a starch, and a sugary, empty one at that.

I understand food aversions. Me and cheese have never gotten along. Although I do not eat a lot of dairy, it is not the taste of dairy that bothers me, but the taste of *old* dairy, whether it has gone bad in my milk jug or has been allowed to age into cheese, cottage cheese, sour cream, curds or yogurt. For years I despised the taste of butter, too.

But I quit saying I hated these things—especially cheese—when I realized how many cheeses are actually in foods I love. It gives substance to any good casserole and holds together all the toppings on my (g-free) pizzas. There are more than nine hundred known cheeses in the world; I have found two mild ones that, in moderation (three or four times a year), agree with me. And I now adore butter. Taste buds do change!

But even if I had not made those changes, I got plenty of calcium from other sources. The same cannot be said for vegetable abstention: The nutrients and antioxidants found in vegetables and fruits are not found in any other food group. Supplements and vitamins alone cannot deliver them either.

A diet of only meat and carbs robs your body of the ability to produce antioxidants, which fight cancer, and packs on fat that becomes harder and harder to lose as you age, especially "visceral fat." According to an article entitled "The Truth about Fat" published on WebMD.com,

> Visceral or "deep" fat wraps around the inner organs and spells trouble for your health. How do you know if you have it? "If you have a large waist or belly, of course you have visceral fat," the author, Whitmer says. Visceral fat drives up your risk for diabetes, heart disease, stroke, and even dementia.[4]

The Veggie-Hater's Prayer

Do not be a vegetable bigot. Live a little! Or live a lot and extend your life. Pray this prayer with me if you need help liking vegetables and fruits, or if you want to begin liking more of them:

God, I see from Your Word that You gave me vegetables and fruits as food. I want what You want for me. I will not allow those dots on my tongue—my taste buds—to rule my life or determine how long I live. Change my palate,

Lord, and help me begin to eat vegetables and fruits. I will do it by faith, God. But help me enjoy it. I lay aside my prejudice about vegetables and fruits and ask You to help me make better choices for a longer life. Color my plate, Lord. Amen.

Prepare to Make Changes

You are about to undo years of pollution from processed foods, tap water toxins and even poisons from household cleaners. Have you ever considered what is in your shampoo? What about your lotions? Your skin is your body's largest organ, so it would serve you well to start reading labels. There are plenty of good alternatives out there for household cleaners and beauty products! Now is the time to do a little online research and bring healing to your body.

Keep in mind that any time you are downwind from a pollutant—whether it be from the car exhaust in front of you or the secondhand smoke from a friend's cigarette or strong cleaning chemicals in your pantry—your body has to process those toxins. I remember one time (prepare yourself for graphic) I was seated in the back of an airplane and for the whole trip smelled a horrific, chemical odor. Perhaps it was from the lavatory or perhaps it was something else in the pressurized cabin air, but I could not wait to get off that plane.

Finally I did and . . . deep breath . . . ah! I could finally flush out my lungs. But then, when I was using the restroom the next day, about eighteen hours after I had gotten off that plane, there was that smell again. So what had processed the chemicals? My kidneys! Probably my lungs and liver, too. But since urine is what was exiting my body, that is what the chemicals jumped into. It is interesting how long those chemicals stayed in me and how long it took my organs to process them before they exited.

And how did the chemicals actually get into my body to begin with? Through my nose with every breath and through every pore of my skin. Crazy.

And do not forget other odors that are so familiar you do not give their toxicity another thought. Ever stepped into a beauty salon and caught that first whiff of hair spray, fingernail polish remover and perm and colorant chemicals? You are so excited about your nearing physical transformation that you cannot even hear your internal organs screaming out for backup! Always remember to visit salons first thing in the morning before such toxins have a chance to accumulate for the day. Meanwhile, thank God for your body's filters: the liver, kidneys, skin and more. God created them to filter toxins, and that is exactly what they do. So *that is* what we will be cleaning during the next thirty days. All your filters. We are going to pamper them and say thanks for all their hard work.

Prepare Your Bath

Of utmost important is *how* you usher these toxins out of your body. Dredging them up is one thing, but getting rid of them is another. You cannot expect your bladder and bowels to do all the work.

Remember that your skin is your body's largest organ and can be most effective in the detox process. One of the least expensive ways to expel the toxins is through baths in Epsom salts. Epsom salts are pure magnesium sulfate; I choose those that have some essential oils—fragrant, natural oils—in them. A fifteen-minute soak does the trick, drawing out toxins and letting them go right down the drain.

Use one pound of salts per bath. It usually comes in three-pound bags, comprising three baths. This will last you one week. (Yes, you just got permission to take three long, hot soaks a week. So tell everyone you are off-limits then.) You may wish to use plain Epsom salts and just sprinkle in the essential oils of your choice as you are getting into the tub and after the water has been turned off.

The best oils for detoxing are lavender, geranium, basil, lemon, grapefruit, peppermint and rosemary. I have tried them all, and often in combination. Make sure you use a certified medical grade essential oil and not a cheap aromatic oil. There is healing power in the oils of the plants God made, and you want the real deal when purging toxins from your system. You can use these same oils in a massage with a "carrier oil" (olive oil, grapeseed or fractionated coconut oil), whether you get someone at home to do the massaging or carry them to your massage therapist.

Prepare Your Skin

Another great detox aid is skin brushing. Never heard of it? It takes only about five minutes and is both soothing and stimulating. There are tremendous health benefits, too, because one-third of the toxins in your body are removed through your skin. Here are the basic steps.

Use a long-handled, natural (not synthetic) bristle brush, such as horsehair. Remove clothing and stand in the shower with water turned off. It will be easy to rinse away the dead skin and toxins you brush off. Start at your feet and in long, sweeping motions brush upward. Always brush toward your heart to improve circulation.

As you brush, prayerfully say good-bye to all the toxins God is removing from your spirit and mind, not just your body. Are there certain people who have gotten "under your skin"? Now would be a good time to forgive and turn these people over to God. As long as you are standing still for five minutes you might as well multitask and spend the time in prayer.

When you have finished, rinse off in warm water. The pores of your skin are now open and will soak up anything you put on them, so do not use harsh soaps. Gently dry off and apply a natural oil, such as coconut oil or olive oil, and feel free to add a drop of your favorite essential oil.

Brush your body often. Daily, if you are experiencing heavy detox symptoms (and those symptoms are spelled out in a moment under "Prepare for Physical Side Effects"). Try it for these thirty days and you will notice an increased glow and smoothness in your skin.

You might want to invest in an infrared portable sauna. Not steam and not just plain electric, but infrared, which is the only type of sauna that can heat the body at its core cellular level for a deep, cleansing sweat. Portable and stationary units of various makes and sizes are available in a wide price range online. (I found mine on eBay for $150.)

Sweating is a safe and phenomenal way to remove bodily toxins quickly. Infrared saunas stimulate collagen production, have anti-aging and skin purification abilities and are just plain relaxing. By the way, do not get overwhelmed at the thought of any investment purchases I am suggesting. They will unarguably boost the effects of this thirty-day detox with visible results, but they are not mandatory. Save up and add them as you can.

With all this skin brushing and, if possible, sauna use, do not forget to change your sheets every few days, washing them in very hot water. This is important since one third of all toxins exit the body through your skin.

Prepare Your Schedule

I want you to think of the next thirty days as sacred. They are an investment in the rest of your life, so approach them seriously. If you have a crazy, busy month ahead, you probably need to wait. Nobody can take a thirty-day vacation and focus entirely on him or herself (that is more like rehab). But do make sure you can spend more time in prayer, more time in reflection and more time in the kitchen. And, hey, if you need rehab, go for it and take me along! I am with you in spirit.

The thirty days do not have to be an exact calendar month either, like March or May. Perhaps you could treat yourself to a spirit, mind and body birthday present and plan the detox to end the day before your birthday. Give yourself the gift of a better you. Just make sure you earmark your thirty days consecutively. The detoxes are designed in layers to achieve an optimum total body cleanse, and doing them out of order or going back to your regular diet in between will preempt the goal of the entire detox.

Also consider your social calendar before you start this detox. Look ahead to birthday parties, anniversaries, church socials, dinners out, family reunions and more. You need to get a game plan for how you are going to stick to the program and not compromise your results.

If you are invited out for a meal, ask instead to grab coffee (decaf), tea (the honey and lemon are good for you) or a naturally sweetened smoothie (bonus points!). For in-home invitations you can always bring a thermos of your own detox soup or, better yet, invite your friends to your house and prepare an entrée from this book. Lead by example!

Consider getting an accountability partner for the thirty days. Your friend might want his or her own book to be able to follow along more specifically with what you are doing—sharing the devotionals, etc. Stop and think: Who might want to support you during this special month? And who needs *your* support for his or her own faith transformation?

Bottom line is that those closest to you need to know you are following *The 30-Day Faith Detox*. It will be a beautiful way for you to share with others what God is doing in you spirit, mind and body. And you never know: You might just inspire others to jump onboard.

Prepare for Physical Side Effects

Let's be smart and look at some of the symptoms that can arise from detoxing. This detox is unique because we will be purifying your body, mind, spirit (and thus, faith). There will be reverberations in each. First, we will look at the physical indicators that will let you know you are detoxing effectively.

When you begin the process of excluding certain foods from your diet and including others, your body will start eliminating toxins. How? In creative ways you might not have thought of. True, there is bowel elimination, but these toxins will be looking for other means of escape, including through your liver, kidneys and the pores of your skin. Your body will become fixated on saying good-bye to these toxins. The longer that good-bye takes, or the longer their journey is out of your body (depending on how much has built up), the more you might feel a little under the weather as all that "rubbish" leaves your system.

Have you ever dusted and swept a room or a garage that has been closed off for a long while? Everything gets stirred up and after just a couple of breaths you are sneezing from the dirt and dust that is entering your body. (Actually, the sneezing is preventing it from entering to begin with.) You might even have to wear a mask. But once all the dust is gone, the air becomes clear again, the mask can come off and the sneezing stops. The room is clean!

Well, think of your bodily detox in the same way. You may have physical reactions as the "dust and dirt" are leaving your body, but they will not last long. And you will feel so much better once they are all gone. Press through the symptoms. Let's take a look at what they might be:

- Changes in bowel movements
- Bloating, tummy ache
- Skin changes, breakouts
- Headaches or malaise
- Fatigue
- Changes in sleep or dreams
- Food cravings
- Chills
- Congestion, feeling as if a cold is coming on
- Feeling irritable or grumpy

Now that I have thoroughly scared you, let me remind you: This is withdrawal! But you can do it because you are worth it. Besides, some people experience few or no symptoms at all. I hardly experienced any. If you do, remember Epsom salt baths, skin-brushing, daily water quotas and infrared sauna time.

Now let me comfort you by telling you some of the benefits of detoxing:

- Weight loss
- Increased energy
- Brighter, clearer skin
- Better breath
- Clearer thinking
- Bowel regularity
- Healthier hair
- Lifted depression
- Clearer sinuses
- Stronger immune system

Another piece of good news for you is that with my detox program, there is no need to "break the detox" afterward, meaning ease yourself back on to normal food. You will be eating normal food the entire time! My goal here is that by the end of the thirty days you will have learned a "new normal," and will have set new standards and patterns that you can continue with on Day 31 and beyond.

Prepare for Spirit and Soul Side Effects

Just as you will experience some mild physical symptoms that let you know you are on the right cleansing track, so you will experience some spiritual and emotional side effects. They, too, will confirm that you are progressing.

Remember: The enemy does not want you healed. He does not want you whole. He wants you to be unclean. His ambition for your life is to make sure you are emotionally crippled, physically toxic and spiritually bankrupt. And you are about to dash his ambitions. You need to expect him to be angry. He will put up a fight. But guess what? You will win. You will recognize his temper tantrums and not give in.

What do his temper tantrums feel like? Well, you might confuse them with your own emotions. During this detox you might experience a heightened sense of your feelings and the way you process responses. Do not be influenced by Satan's reactions. Resist the temptation to surrender to bitterness, anger, discontentment and offense—but do expect to have brushes with them. If a certain devotional requires you to forgive someone, you might think, *I will never forgive her!* But in that moment, you will remember not to give in to the enemy. That is Satan's reaction, not yours. Yours is the same as Jesus', who taught us to pray that God will "forgive us our sins as we forgive those who sin against us."

Remember, too, that with each day's devotional you will be bringing all sorts of memories to the surface. With them will come a bevy of emotions. This is why it is extra important for you to spend additional time in prayer this month. Just as drinking extra water is important for proper bodily elimination, so spending extra time in prayer and drinking in the Holy Spirit is crucial for your spiritual and emotional cleansing.

The results are going to be fantastic. You can expect eventually to hit your stride and recognize God's voice as never before. Your instincts will become laser-sharp, and your discernment intensely acute. Whereas the emotional detoxing will cause you to experience some lows, the spiritual detoxing will cause you to experience some powerful highs. Get ready to experience God in new ways! Prepare to be amazed!

Here is my prayer for you: "Now may the God of peace himself sanctify you completely, and may your whole spirit and soul and body be kept blameless at the coming of our Lord Jesus Christ" (1 Thessalonians 5:23).

SECTION 3

Social Influence Toxins

Spiritual Emphasis: Taking control over worldly appetites and unhealthy environments while eliminating the ingested social influences that infect your faith

Emotions Associated with These Toxins: agitation, fear, stress, confusion, rebellion, dissatisfaction, doubt, shame, guilt, rejection, depression, grief, anger, judgment, abandonment, isolation

Bodily Systems Detoxed:
> Days 1 and 2: Digestive (mouth, esophagus, stomach, liver, large intestines)
> Days 3 and 4: Excretory (small intestines, colon, rectum)
> Days 5 and 6: Urinary (kidneys, bladder, gallbladder)

Section Colors

Besides the specified greens, this section's support color is *yellow*. This color's fresh vegetables and fruits contain carotenoids, which, acting as antioxidants, protect cells from free radicals. What are antioxidants and free radicals? In a nutshell, free radicals are the bad guys and antioxidants are the good guys. The more good guys you have on hand when the bad guys show up, the less likely they are to set up camp and spread disease. The good guys get their ammo from nutrients in the foods we eat, and the bad guys get theirs from pollution, sunlight, radiation, cigarette smoke and stress. No one is exempt from the battle with the radical bad guys. The only way to keep them at bay is to eat foods that are filled with the good guys, our heroes, the antioxidants.

The carotenoid family consists of smaller families of pigments called carotenes and xanthophylls. Carotenoids are precursors to vitamin A, meaning they can be transformed into vitamin A through metabolic reaction. Carotenoids are particularly prized in the digestive tract, which stretches into the excretory tract. Vitamin A helps grow epithelial cells, the type of cells that comprise the intestinal tract lining. Mature epithelial cells form the strongest barrier there.

The detox recipes for Days 1–6 will cleanse, among many other things, the liver and kidneys. These are important filters for everything that circulates throughout your entire body and then exits it, so it is very important that this system be cleansed first, since it will champion the detoxification of the rest of your body in the next thirty days. Menus are provided each day. All recipes are included in the recipe section at the back of the book, as well as preparation ideas for your dinner meal, since that meal could be prepared in many different ways. You get to choose!

Note that in this grocery list I chose green, or less ripe, bananas over yellow (both have white meat), since the more yellow a banana, the more sugar it contains. This trade is not only a better option for trimming belly fat during this digestive system detox, but it also helps those with kidney issues, especially when related to diabetes.

If you are a kidney patient, please note: While yellow potassium-rich produce is very beneficial for kidneys, if you are on dialysis or have kidney issues seek advice from your doctor or nutritionist before consuming extra amounts of potassium (i.e., mango, spinach, zucchini, potato, yogurt, avocado, salmon and bananas).[1]

Section Grocery List

Purchase one or two of each of the following fruits and vegetables, depending on your appetite level. If the fruit or vegetable is tiny, purchase enough for at least two cups. In the case of leaf vegetables, one head, bunch or bag of each variety mentioned will suffice. You may also double up on one vegetable or fruit if you dislike another, but be open to trying new things! With each section you will better be able to gauge your appetite and adjust your purchases to accommodate it.

Yellows	yellow pepper, yellow potato, yellow squash, yellow onion, lemon, pineapple, yellow apples, applesauce, mango
Greens	endive, romaine, spinach, cucumber, celery, watercress, green cabbage, zucchini, avocado, kiwi, green (less ripe) banana
Allowed Additions	quinoa, brown rice; fresh cranberries, black beans, garbanzo beans, eggs; oils: olive, coconut and/or flaxseed; chicken broth; once or twice a week you may trade your veggie snack for a shake (see Recipes)
Herb/Spice Options	turmeric, cumin, ginger, goldenseal, mint leaves, parsley
Tea	dandelion, milk thistle (see Recipes); booster option: decaf green tea; for flavor add an extra bag of any caffeine-free fruit or berry tea

Optional Meat	only vegetables are recommended, but a three-ounce serving of organic poultry or fish (size of deck of cards) is permitted at dinner
Nuts	almonds, cashews, walnuts
Water	drink half your body weight in ounces daily
Bases for Smoothies	choice of milks: organic 2%, unsweetened almond, coconut; choice of waters: coconut, aloe
Rest	nine hours nightly

DAY 1

Spiritual Toxin: Media and Your Mind

You wake up one morning to an annoying ringtone alarm on your phone that you did not know you had, not that you slept much after that violent, R-rated action flick. You roll out of bed with breakfast in mind and turn on the television for some morning news, instantly bombarded with images of scantily clad models ill-placed for their time slot. You turn off the television after the news gets too depressing and you have lost your appetite for breakfast, deciding to get your news online today. But before you can read even one headline, half-a-dozen pop-ups sneak past your Internet filters and insist that you go on a certain celebrity diet, warn you to stop eating a certain three freak foods that are making you fat and creepily remind you about that item you left in an online shopping cart three days ago, luring you to come back and buy it.

You shut down your computer and head to work. You turn on the car radio and hear Linda Ronstadt telling you you're no good. You flip to talk radio, where two political authors are arguing about health care reform at the top of their lungs, joined by an atheist who claims that if there were such a being as "God," which he denies there is, we could determine from the number of sick people in the world that this God does not heal, that He does not even care about mankind and, furthermore, neither do His money-hungry ministers. All of this while passing three billboards of finely dressed pastors inviting you to their mega-churches. But the billboards change every few seconds and prevent you from retaining the information about their homeless ministries so you can prove the atheist wrong.

At work you jump into the elevator, checking social media on your phone on the way up to your nine a.m. staff meeting, only to scroll past four episodes of Facebook venting by disgruntled friends. You try to ignore the magazines in the lobby of your office, which are drama-laden with the latest scandals, but you are pretty sure one of them features the scantily clad model you saw before the breakfast you never had. You realize at that point that she probably never eats breakfast either and wonder if that is the secret to losing your muffin-top. Aaaaand . . . now you suddenly crave muffins. You race into your meeting and take your seat at the conference table. Why do you already need a nap?

"Good morning!" says your boss, but you have not felt good since Linda Ronstadt. You let out a huge sigh, which makes you remember an article you read on "air-hunger" being a sign of needing therapy. Do you need therapy? You decide on the celebrity diet instead.

You do not need a celebrity diet. You need a media diet. The daily visual inundation from television, movies, billboards, magazine print images and social media, coupled with the constant audio pelting of talk radio, syndicated advertisements and musical playlists, has polluted our peace and diluted our faith. That invisible, silent territory where God once had our full attention is now cluttered with competing voices. It is harder and harder to hear God's still, small voice through it all. Romans 10:17 (NKJV) says that "faith comes by hearing and hearing by the word of God." It only makes sense that if we are hearing more of media and less of God, real faith will never "come." Remember:

I will set no worthless thing before my eyes; I hate the work of those who fall away; it shall not fasten its grip on me.

Psalm 101:3 NASB

Finally, brethren, whatever things are true, whatever things are noble, whatever things are just, whatever things are pure, whatever things are lovely, whatever things are of good report, if there is any virtue and if there is anything praiseworthy—meditate on these things. The things which you learned and received and heard and saw in me, these do, and the God of peace will be with you.

Philippians 4:8–9 NKJV

Corresponding Emotional Toxins

People who ingest too much of or the wrong kinds of media or social media are often easily agitated, fearful, stressed and confused. Let's pray now for God to renew your mind and spirit from these potential influences and help you set new standards for yourself that will benefit your faith:

Father God, I ask You to bring to my mind right now those forms of media and social media I ingest that You would like for me to consume less of. God, how much time daily with these things is healthy for me? [Wait and listen.] Trade my morning desire for my devices for a daily devotional time with You. Help me emotionally to eliminate any fear, doubt, confusion and agitation I experience as a result of media gluttony. Show me movie alternatives that will not clog my spirit and defile my faith. And give me the guts to say no to all the rest, no matter the inconvenience it brings. Keep my eyes from unclean things, whether on-line or in print, and bring purity to my thoughts. I allow Your holiness to invade my choices of music, and I give You full permission to convict me about any song on any playlist on any device that I own. Give me grace for this new media diet, Father. In Jesus' name, Amen.

Correlating Physical Detox

Today and tomorrow we cleanse the upper and middle digestive tracts.

It has been said, "You are what you eat," but it could also be said, "You are what you do not digest or eliminate." Another nutritional expression is that "Death begins in the colon," and that is because research reveals that almost all chronic ailments or discomforts have a connection to the digestive tract. Thus, we are going to start this detox by flushing your digestive tract with the Saltwater Lemon Flush. Out with the old and in with the new!

Salt has long been esteemed as a preservative and disinfectant. Just as you would gargle with saltwater for a sore throat, pat salt on an open wound for quicker healing or soak in a salt bath to draw out toxins, so you can count on saltwater flushes to act like a healing bath for the inside of your body. Doing this in the morning has optimum results since the stomach is in an empty, fasting state. This method is much safer (and less costly) than colonic cleanses or enemas, and affects much more than just the colon because it travels through the entire digestive tract (from mouth to rectum).

Today and tomorrow, within thirty minutes of rising, place two teaspoons pink Himalayan salt (but *not* iodized table salt) and two teaspoons lemon juice (which is full of vitamin C and other cleansing nutrients) in a 32-ounce glass of filtered water (*not* tap water). Water should be lukewarm, warmed on the stove and not in a microwave. Drink the mixture as quickly as you can and then go on about your morning. Some nutritionists suggest lying on your right side so the mixture can quickly reach the entrance to the small intestines, but it is my experience that this will happen naturally as you move around and go about your morning.

Within about thirty minutes you will hear tummy rumblings and in another thirty to ninety minutes you will feel the urge to eliminate. You may experience cramping, diarrhea or nausea; this is the stirring of the toxins in preparation for elimination. The 84 vitamins and minerals in the Himalayan pink salt are providing healing and nourishment to your entire intestinal tract, from mouth to rectum, a space that is between twenty and thirty feet long. After you eliminate fully you are free to eat breakfast. (This will likely be one to two hours after drinking the flush.)

Hour Before Breakfast	Saltwater Lemon Flush
Breakfast	The Yummy Tummy Trimmer Smoothie
Mid-a.m. Juicing	Laura's One-Two Punch
Lunch	Sixcess Salad
Snack	snack liberally from your yellows and greens
Dinner	choose one green and one yellow fruit or vegetable (see Recipes for prep ideas); pair with brown rice or quinoa tossed with section spices and section nuts or beans
Nightcap	Detox Tea

Closing Blessing

May God heal your digestive tract of any illnesses and bless your diet during this detox as you seek Him about the elimination of certain media and social media outlets that you are ingesting too much of!

DAY 2

Spiritual Toxin: Ungodly Counsel

I am sure, like me, you love the book of Psalms and have experienced its repeated value in your life. There are 2,461 verses in Psalms (plus 137 unnumbered ones), but if I were to ask you to quote the very first verse from this very famous collection, could you? Here it is: "Blessed is the man that walketh not in the counsel of the ungodly, nor standeth in the way of sinners, nor sitteth in the seat of the scornful" (Psalm 1:1 KJV).

I live in Nashville, Tennessee, also known as Music City, USA. Even though it is home to gospel music and is the birthplace of bluegrass and folk, it is primarily known as the home of country music. Granted, I do not know how many country songs have ever been created nor what all the verses are all about, but I can pretty much guarantee you that the first one ever written did not include advice on staying away from sinners or steering clear of ungodly counsel. In fact I am pretty sure it was quite the opposite. The fact that the very first verse in this Spirit-inspired collection of psalms involves choosing your friends wisely is reason enough for me to recognize God's emphasis on the importance of this spiritual and social truth: *Show me your friends and I will show you your future.*

Look at Psalm 1:1 again. There are three types of people who will derail you from the path God has for you—and you have encountered all of them. Even though you might be tempted to lump them all into one personage, do not, because you need to be on the lookout for all three: (1) the ungodly, (2) sinners and (3) the scornful. What is the difference? They are three separate stages of wickedness but follow somewhat of a progression.

The "ungodly" are those who do not have God. Perhaps they are law-abiding citizens, upstanding in the community, benevolent, kind and quiet, but they make no room for God or His statutes in their lives. In Psalm 1:1 it is the Hebrew word *rasha'* and means "guilty."

"Sinners" are more than just guilty, because guilt can be a public or private thing. Sinners are open offenders, and a little easier to spot. Psalm 1:1 uses the Hebrew word *chatta'* meaning "offender." It implies an ungodly person who has decided to take his ungodly thoughts and turn them into ungodly actions.

The "scornful" are in a different class altogether. They are not just ungodly and not just sinners; they have shaken their fists and raised their voices against heaven. They take pride in mocking, scoffing and spewing hatred toward all things Christian. It is the Hebrew word *luwts* meaning "to be inflated, scoff, boast, mock and deride." This is different from an ungodly person who might keep his opinions to himself. Thus, we can say that all scorners are ungodly but not all the ungodly are scorners. *Luwts* also means "ambassador." Scorners act as if it is their job to speak on behalf of the ungodly, the sinners and those who disdain organized religion altogether.

Let me revisit the subject of country music—not to criticize this thriving industry, but simply to use it as a backdrop for observing these three types. You generally do not see the "scornful" on country music's star roster. The majority of country music artists would never shake their fists at God or mock Him. Perhaps that is because country music has its roots in gospel music or maybe it would lop off a large chunk of their fan base, but, whatever the reason, you just do not hear God-bashing, church-hating country music stars as you do in other music industry genres. In fact, it is quite the opposite. You hear plenty of songs about church, God's love, faith and grace.

In the midst of that, however, compromise abounds in the form of ungodliness and sin that Psalm 1 speaks of. Just listen to some old country tunes or watch an afternoon of country music videos. You will see a Bible in one hand and learn before long that someone else's spouse is holding the other. Jesus is welcome to take the wheel but there is whiskey in the glove box in the next song. So the message seems to be that as long as you are not a scorner, sin and ungodliness is okay. But it is not okay, and according to Psalm 1:1, we are forbidden from doing three things with those who head in those directions: We must not *stand* with them, *sit* with them or *walk* in their counsel. (And needless to say, we also should not lie with them.)

So what does it mean to "walk in the counsel of the ungodly"? Well, first of all, to walk in the counsel of the ungodly as opposed to that of sinners or scorners is dangerous because it can be deceptive. Remember, the ungodly appear to be kind, benevolent law-abiding citizens. They appear to have your best interests in mind. It is easy to take their advice—as worldly as it may be—and think this could be God's will for your life. Their counsel looks enticing and appears to be wise, but in the end, it brings death, not life. Perhaps you are a teenager and a friend is telling you that your parents do not know what is best for you, or maybe you are in an unhappy marriage and a psychologist is telling you it is okay to leave. After all, you deserve to be happy, right?

Ungodly counsel often brings immediate happiness, but no lasting fruit. Your flesh might feel satisfied by being angry at your parents and gratified by leaving your spouse for someone "better," but a real friend or wise counselor is going to tell you to stick it out and not settle for fleeting satisfaction or self-gratification. Doing the right thing is not always the easiest thing, but it comes with the greatest earthly reward (not to mention, heavenly). And in case you are wondering, even the godly can give ungodly counsel. Just look at Job's friends.

So remember Psalm 1:1 and steer clear of (1) the ungodly, (2) sinners and (3) the scornful. You can remember it by the acronym "U.S.S." In the American military system that acronym means "United States Ship," as in the U.S.S. *Constitution*. So just remember never to take a ride on the "U.S.S. *Counsel*" because it is a ship that will take you nowhere!

Other Scriptures to read: Genesis 3:1–24; Jeremiah 7:24; Ephesians 5:11.

Corresponding Emotional Toxins

People who are the recipients of ungodly counsel often suffer from confusion, rebellion, dissatisfaction, stress and doubt. Let's pray now for God to renew your mind and spirit from these potential influences and to help you set new standards for yourself that will benefit your faith:

> *Father God, I want only Your counsel. I do not want it said of me that I settled for anything short of Your wisdom. I need it in my life, relationships, job and health. In Jesus' name I break off the toxic social influence of ungodly counsel from my life! I repent for any time I have taken the easy road and gone against wise counsel. I ask for healing from the confusion, dissatisfaction, stress, rebellion and doubt that it caused others or me. Help me right any wrongs caused by my taking this ungodly counsel. I ask that You give me better discernment the next time. In Jesus' name, Amen.*

Correlating Physical Detox

Today we finish cleansing the upper and middle digestive tracts. Drink the Saltwater Lemon Flush upon rising, per yesterday's instructions. Repeat yesterday's meal plan, experimenting with this section's colors.

Closing Blessing

May God heal your digestive tract of any ailments and bless your cleansing as you seek Him about ridding your life of ungodly counsel.

DAY 3

Spiritual Toxin: The Ties That Bind (Breaking Soul-Ties)

What even is a soul? Is it the same thing as your spirit? Does it go to heaven one day, or is that what your spirit is for? Since the word *soul* is used so often to mean so many things, before we discuss one of its most pervasive toxins we need to distinguish it from *spirit*.

First, listen to this Scripture that supports the fact that the soul and spirit are separate: "The word of God is living and active, sharper than any two-edged sword, piercing to the division of soul and of spirit, of joints and of marrow, and discerning the thoughts and intentions of the heart" (Hebrews 4:12). So if the soul and spirit can be divided, then let's look at what they mean in the Greek, which is what Hebrews 4:12 was written in.

Soul is a translation of *psyche*, which, among many things, means "the force that animates the body and shows itself in breathing; the seat of the feelings, desires, affections, aversions; the (human) soul in so far as it is constituted that by the right use of the aids offered it by God it can attain its highest end and secure eternal blessedness; the soul regarded as a moral being designed for everlasting life; the soul as an essence that differs from the body and is not dissolved by death (distinguished from other parts of the body)."

Spirit or *pneuma* among other things means "the vital principal by which the body is animated; the source by which the human being feels, thinks, desires, decides and acts; a simple essence, devoid of matter; a human soul that has left the body; the efficient source of any power."

Perhaps you have heard that the soul is merely the "mind, will and emotions," and that the spirit is that which is eternal. *Psyche* is the word from which we get our English word *psychology*, and that seems to drive a sharper wedge between the two, reducing "soul" to something entirely temporal while "spirit" is seemingly elevated to that which is eternal.

It is, however, a bit more miraculous than that. They are actually very similar, but with a marked difference. Let's compare the definitions again. Both "animate" the body, "feel," "desire" and have "affections." And it also appears that both are eternal, since the definition for soul includes: "it can attain its highest end and secure *eternal* blessedness, the soul regarded as a moral being designed for *everlasting life;* the soul as an essence that differs from the body and *is not dissolved by death*."

This is precious because it reveals that our souls will be intact in heaven, too. In other words, we will have our same personalities and affections. How fun!

But there is a difference: "Spirit" is defined as including a soul but "soul" is not defined as including a spirit. To be more specific, "spirit" is "a soul that has left the body" (*spirit, pneuma*: "a human soul that has left the body, the efficient source . . ."). But your soul never sources or contains your spirit. So on earth, the two are separate and very much in need of distinct stewardship. Your spirit cannot have a "spirit-tie" but your soul can have a "soul-tie." So let's now discuss where that is found in Scripture, how you can tell if it has happened to you and what you can do about it.

A soul-tie is a past or present unrestrained emotional state, occurring in human relationships, that affects and interferes with your relationship with God. It involves excessive loyalty or even codependency, although sometimes the dependency is not mutual. It is like an addiction, except instead of being tied to a substance or object, the addiction is to a person.

This can occur between friends, fans and celebrities, gang or club leaders and their members, drug users, drinking buddies, parents and children, or other relatives. Sometimes souls get tied together in settings that seem harmless—for example, war survivors or trauma victims who congregate to relive the past or because they rely on one another to get through life.

Soul-ties involve a disproportionate focus on someone from the past or present, but it does not have to be carried into your future!

Look at Deuteronomy 13:6 for an example of two souls being tied together for an ungodly purpose: "If your brother, the son of your mother, or your son or your daughter or the wife you embrace or your friend who is as your own soul entices you secretly saying, 'Let us go and serve other gods' . . ."

Did you catch that telling definition? "Your friend *who is as your own soul*." Here the Hebrew word for *soul* is *nephesh*, meaning (among other things) "soul, passion, the seat of appetites, activity of the mind, activity of the will, emotion."

Another place where soul-ties occur most often is within sexual relationships. Mark 10 explains that God made male and a female who join in marriage, unite and become "one flesh." But this "one flesh" connection occurs even if the two are not husband and wife. Listen to Paul in 1 Corinthians 6:16: "Do you not know that he who is joined to a prostitute becomes one body with her? For, as it is written, 'The two will become one flesh.'"

We see another example of an ungodly soul-tie in Genesis 34:8: "But Hamor spoke with them, saying, 'The soul of my son Shechem longs for your daughter. Please give her to him to be his wife.'" Several translations say either "his soul cleaves to your daughter" or "his soul is joined to your daughter." Longing, cleaving or joining, it does not matter; all three indicate a soul that is tied wrongly to another.

Sexual relations involve the exchange of bodily fluids, which is a powerful union. Those in the occult know this and apply it to their dark rituals involving blood, urine, feces, semen (and more). But their counterfeit usage does not undo the original purpose for this beautiful biblical truth, which was to unite two people into "one flesh."

Almost twenty years ago, a woman asked me to come pray with her in the privacy of her home. She began by expressing to me that she felt marital dissatisfaction. As we began to pray, she confessed something unthinkable to me. She admitted that she had slept with about a hundred men before her current marriage. Having only ever been with one man, I could not fathom such a lifestyle. My heart ached for her as she fell over into my lap and cried in utter brokenness.

She was now married to a successful, godly man, who was aware of her past, and they had wonderful children. It soon became evident to me that her dissatisfaction was not dissatisfaction at all, for she had nothing to be dissatisfied about. Instead, she was experiencing the burdensome bondage of a soul-tie. One hundred soul-ties, in fact.

I did not really know what to pray because the prayers about her dissatisfaction were no longer the issue. Instinctively I began comforting her, ministering grace and mercy to her. As I did this, I heard the Lord tell me to start counting. Not understanding, but with her still in my lap and with my arms around her, I proceeded very slowly: "One . . . two . . . three . . ." The longer and higher I counted, she and I both became aware that the Lord was numbering the men and setting her free from each soul-tie, severing the demonic confusion from having become "one flesh" with so many people.

Sometimes I would get to a certain number and she would burst into tears. Although I am sure she could not remember who "number 42" or "number 65" or "number 93" was, God did, and you could tell from her reaction each time that He was delivering her from the unhealthy affiliation that particular encounter had bred. And what if each of those one hundred men had slept with one hundred women? Unlikely, perhaps, but what if they had slept with five or ten? She would have been tied to those individuals as well. We broke an untold number of soul-ties that day.

When we finished, the woman sat up, dried her tears and thanked me. I am telling you, she was free! It was a glorious experience that I will never forget. I greatly admire this couple, and they are still married today, thanks be to God.

I once read an article online that argued against the existence of soul-ties because the Bible never uses that actual wording. It was very frustrating to me because I have seen with my own eyes the "befores and afters." Plus, there are many English phrases we have come up with in Christendom that are not found in the original Greek or Hebrew; these phrases are usually built around concepts that are very much present in Scripture. Either way, I can only pray that someone bound in the chains of a soul-tie never stumbles across such a compassionless commentary and fails to receive the freedom he or she needs.

If you or someone you know is suffering from an ungodly soul-tie, you (or they) can break it by praying the prayer on the next page. It would also be wise to get rid of anything in your possession that links you to that person (or people). Old photographs, clothing, gifts, etc. God will show you, but you will definitely need to be obedient. (Obviously, if that relationship gained you a child, you cannot get rid of the child. Rather, look at the child as a beautiful redemptive gift from God.)

Once you pray this prayer and "clean house," you will feel the difference, soul and spirit.

Again, the definitions of *soul* and *spirit* are so similar that some see no distinction at all; thus, they believe in the "dichotomy of man," meaning they believe that there are only two parts to man and that the soul and spirit are one.

I am a trichotomist, though, since Scripture says we are made in God's image and God is three Persons. He is Holy Trinity, and we are an "earthly trinity," meaning only that we mirror His divine nature here on earth. Three in one, but separate, nonetheless.

Paul echoes this: "Now may the God of peace himself sanctify you completely, and may your whole spirit and soul and body be kept blameless at the coming of our Lord Jesus Christ" (1 Thessalonians 5:23).

Other Scriptures to meditate on: Ezekiel 13:18–22; 1 Corinthians 6:18.

Corresponding Emotional Toxins

People who have developed soul-ties often experience the toxic emotions of shame, guilt, rejection, dissatisfaction and depression. Let's pray now for God to renew your mind from these potential influences and to help you set new standards for yourself that will benefit your faith:

Father God, I repent for the times I have put another before You. I ask You to break off any soul-ties in Jesus' name. I receive healing from any resulting shame, guilt, rejection, dissatisfaction or depression. I give to You every relationship and memory that is fixated upon the wrong source. I confess that You are my source, God. I will give no excessive loyalty to anyone but You. I ask You to show me any people with whom I am to be in proper, godly covenant, and may those be relationships worthy of Your blessing. In Jesus' name, Amen.

Correlating Physical Detox

Today and tomorrow we cleanse the excretory system.

Breakfast	Bottoms Up Detox Smoothie
Mid-a.m. Juicing	Four-of-a-Kind Juice
Lunch	Take-Five Stir Fry
Snack	snack liberally from your yellows
Dinner	choose one green and one yellow fruit or vegetable (see Recipes for prep ideas); pair with brown rice or quinoa tossed with section spices and section nuts or beans
Nightcap	Detox Tea

Closing Blessing

May God heal your excretory system of any blockages that prevent elimination and bless your detox as you seek Him about the elimination of any soul-ties in your life.

DAY 4

Spiritual Toxin: When Heroes Fall

You know that moment when you realize a person you look up to is actually human? We all hate those moments. But life is full of them.

Today's devotional comes with a warning: It may summon emotions and memories you were not bargaining for when you cracked open this book today. It is, however, the only effective way I can think of to convey the gut-wrenching grief of losing a role model. Since you just might be one yourself one day (or are already), I urge you to keep reading.

So where were you when you found out about Bill Clinton's adulterous activities, perjury and impeachment? (I still have his national video confession on VHS and refuse to trash it.) Or going back a few more years, how did you feel when you watched Richard Nixon's resignation over Watergate? What about when you found out about Arnold Schwarzenegger's affair and love child? And what feelings do the following names bring to mind? Michael Jackson, Stephen Collins, Anthony Weiner, John Edwards, Britney Spears, etc.? Remember those cringeworthy mug shots of celebs like Lindsay Lohan, Mel Gibson, Glen Campbell, Amanda Bynes, Jane Fonda, Randy Travis and Yasmine Bleeth? And for you sports fans, how do you feel when you hear the names Lance Armstrong, Jerry Sandusky, Michael Vick, Tiger Woods, Steve McNair, Pete Rose, Sammy Sosa, Mark McGwire, Tonya Harding, Barry Bonds or Roger Clemens? Or what about the heart-rending suicides (intentional or unintentional) of Robin Williams, Whitney Houston, Kurt Cobain, Marilyn Monroe and Philip Seymour Hoffman? I did not even know until doing this study that Vincent van Gogh, Mark Antony and Tchaikovsky committed suicide. I guess heroes have been falling for a long time.

But as sickened and unsettled as you might have been after hearing about these heroes' crestfallen endings, somehow it is worse when it is a religious hero who transgresses. They are not supposed to fall, right?

Ted Haggard, Jim Bakker, Jimmy Swaggart, Robert Tilton, Cardinal Bernard Law, on and on the list goes. Some ministers wound up in the Televangelist Hall of Shame for sexual sin, and others turned into Daddy "Morebucks" and wasted their donors' monies. But what about Judas' betrayal of Jesus? What about how the Israelites felt when their courageous leader, Moses, was forbidden by God from entering into the Promised Land over that rock and water incident? What about David committing murder and adultery as king? Talk about scandalous.

But there is a difference between a baseball player using illegal steroids and your pastor falling into sexual sin. That third-baseman was not responsible to shepherd your soul. He was not training you up into righteousness and purity. Your pastor was. When your pastor falls, a piece of your heart falls with him.

So why do they fall? How can someone who is spiritually on top of the world sink so low? Disconnection? Perhaps. Pride? Yes. Seducing spirits? Bingo. But the seducing spirits only have access to someone who is disconnected and proud, so it becomes a predictable cycle. Paul prophesied that many in the last days will fall away from the faith as a result of demonic, seducing spirits: "Now the Spirit speaketh expressly, that in the latter times some shall depart from the faith, giving heed to seducing spirits, and doctrines of devils" (1 Timothy 4:1 KJV).

Can falling be prevented? Oh, yes. All of us must stay connected to the Body of Christ through regular congregational attendance (see Hebrews 10:25), stay small in our own eyes (see 1 Samuel 15:17–23), develop a disciplined prayer life (see 1 Thessalonians 5:17) and do away with all relationships that will bring us down: "Do not be misled: 'Bad company corrupts good character'" (1 Corinthians 15:33 NIV). Spiritual stability *is* conditional.

A few years ago, I wrote a hero list—the top fifteen influencers who intersected with my life and changed its course drastically for the better, making me what I am today. But guess what? When I revisited that list today I saw that of the fifteen, twelve have failed me in some significant way over time, and of those twelve, eight flat out hurt me (most not intentionally).

Of the fifteen, only three have never hurt or disappointed me. Three! And what did those three have in common? That I did not actually spend a lot of one-on-one time with them. I am sure that if I had they would have had the shining opportunity to fail me, too. That is life! That *is* the beauty of life! There is no progress without risk, and relationships are full of them.

The other reason we sometimes lose heart and waver emotionally when a hero falls is because it puts its finger on something in all of us that is capable of causing us to lose footing and take our own nosedive. Scripture is clear that not one of us is righteous—not one—and all fall short of the glory of God. And let's not forget 1 Corinthians 10:12 (NIV): "If you think you are standing firm, be careful that you don't fall!"

Perhaps someone let you down. How should you respond? Well, Romans 15:1–2 says, "We who are strong have an obligation to bear with the failings of the weak, and not to please ourselves. Let each of us please his neighbor for his good, to build him up." I love verse 2 in the Weymouth New Testament: "We should help others do what is right and build them up in the Lord."

I have had spiritual heroes fall near me before. Some fell so quietly that, like that tree in the forest, hardly anyone noticed at first. Others fell so hard that those of us watching had to scatter to stay safe from the splintering, the impact and the quaking ground. Sometimes the aftershocks are so great that your heart does not even have time to miss the once-towering tree, but then moments come of looking back and missing the shadow it once cast.

If this has happened to you, this is the very place where you have a choice: Become bitter and judgmental, or grow and start casting your own shadow.

About twenty or so years into our marriage, Chris and I had several friends who suddenly started divorcing. It was distressing to watch these longtime friends with longtime marriages and multiple children be torn apart. Our kids had all grown up together. It was especially difficult to watch many of the "divorced children" lose their faith in God. After several of these divorces, one of our sons had a friend over for the night. He was one whose parents had stayed together through all of this turmoil. He said to me, "Mrs. Laura, this has really been hard watching all my friends' parents getting divorced, but I am telling you, if you and Mr. Chris ever got divorced, I would question everything I have ever believed about God, and I think a lot of other people would too."

Wow! That hit my heart hard. What an honor though! Most people have to do something to be a hero. I had only *not* to do something: not get divorced. I realized that something as simple as staying the course can make you a hero.

Say what you will about televangelist Jimmy Swaggart. I never saw the picture of him outside that hotel room in 1988, and I do not care to. All I want to remember about him is that when I was ten years old I heard him singing on television, and his sincerity brought tears to my eyes. I was so moved that I sat down and wrote him a letter, and he wrote me back. He told me that I had cried because the Holy Spirit was drawing me to Himself, and that I needed to give Him my heart. So I did. A few weeks later I walked an aisle at a Baptist church, and I have been serving God ever since. Although my parents had taken me to church and exposed me to Christianity my whole life, it was not until I heard Jimmy Swaggart sing that I experienced the anointing, and that anointing drew me in. I am still here today.

When he fell, did it mean I fell with him? No, of course not. But so often when our heroes fall, we give ourselves an excuse to tumble, falling right into our own evils, hidden and seen. When he fell, did his wife fall too? No, she stuck around and they have been married for more than sixty years now. They are both still in ministry, but I think their greatest ministry has been staying married for six decades through all the public drama.

And say what you will about Josh Duggar and the regrettable events of the spring and summer of 2015, but he is not beyond forgiveness or redemption. I have met Jim Bob and Michelle, and they seem to be genuine folks. Can the family ever regain their footing with the public? From just one brief encounter with them, I can tell you that their main concern is their family and not "the public." They are *still* a family, and God is *still* the God of second and third chances. Only He can redeem the entire saga and turn it for His good. God is far from done using the extraordinary Duggar family with all of their admitted scars, and He is far from done using yours and mine with all of ours. Aren't you glad?

A longtime friend of mine and spiritual mama, Donna Svolto, recently said to me, "Laura, do you know what the Lord told me this morning about Satan falling like lightning from heaven? He said that if one-third of the angels could be deceived by Satan into rebelling against God while they were standing there in His very presence in heaven, then *none of us* down here are beyond being deceived or falling." How remarkably and soberingly true.

I wish no one ever fell, but since Satan fell like lightning from heaven, he has been trying to drag others down with him. Especially spiritual heroes. Some will live in the mud and others will come clean. I deeply respect and admire repenting heroes who stand back up and embrace vulnerable restoration.

I think that makes them superheroes.

Corresponding Emotional Toxins

People whose heroes fall often experience the emotions of grief, anger, judgment and embarrassment. Let's pray now for God to renew your mind and spirit from these potential influences and help you recover:

Father God, I give You my disillusionment and pain. I lift up _____ to You right now and ask You to restore them to You. Forgive them for what they did, how they fell, and heal those it hurt. I release them to You for good. Now, God, patch up my heart wherever it still mourns with grief, anger, judgment and embarrassment. I forgive them entirely and ask You to set my mind free to remember the good they once brought into my life. Thank You for how You have forgiven me before, Lord. You are the God of second chances. In Jesus' name, Amen.

Correlating Physical Detox

Today we finish cleansing the excretory system. Repeat yesterday's meal plan, experimenting with this section's colors.

Closing Blessing

May God cleanse your excretory system of any blockages and toxins as you ask Him to help you process and eliminate any wounds in your life from heroes who have fallen and failed you.

DAY 5

Spiritual Toxin: Divide and Conquer (Church Hits and Splits)

How many churches have you been part of in your entire adult life? And why did you leave each one? If you are over the age of forty and have been in any fewer then four, you are a minority. Me? Three churches. Including the one Chris and I now pastor at Eastgate.

In the first church, we started out in children's ministry as volunteers. We had one child and were quite young ourselves. I started a Christian Dinner Theatre in that church, and by the end of our seven amazing years there, we were both serving in the youth ministry and Chris was an ordained deacon.

Why did we leave? One reason only—since we found no fault in the church, its leaders, pastor, programs or our countless friends there—and that is that we wanted more of the Holy Spirit and wanted home group ministry. So did the then-pastor, but it was a complicated uphill battle in that established, eighty-year-old church. It is still thriving and has passed the one-hundred-year mark. Many of our dearest friends are still there.

Although it felt like tearing off a limb, we and our four young children left for a brand-new church that an older established Nashville congregation had launched. There we found the Holy Spirit moving powerfully in small home groups, as well as in the corporate services. I started a drama department immediately and, before the year was out, we found ourselves in home group ministry as interns. When that group "multiplied" (you never say "divided"), we got our own group and became "cell" leaders. When that group multiplied into three groups, we got our own "zone" and became zone leaders. Once that zone's cells began multiplying, we became district pastors. Along the way, Chris became an ordained elder, and I was ordained as a prophetic teacher. They were ten of the happiest years of our lives.

So what happened? That second church took a real hit that ended in total disillusionment. What was once a 650-member and near-million-dollar-a-year ministry simply disappeared. It was the hardest thing we had ever encountered in our then-twenty-year marriage, and to be honest, I think even now, ten years later, it is still the hardest thing. We were all tangled up in the lives of the members of that church. Our children were all being born together as the years went by; Chris and I had two kids there. We were a fruitful bunch; somebody was always either pregnant or throwing someone else a baby shower. We all gave our youths to that church, to the Lord and to each other.

It has taken ten years and a lot of hard work for members to reconcile with one another because of the events of the church's death. So much work, in fact, that I have to be very careful how I handle the writing of today's devotional. But I have decided to include this story because of how much I wish I had had something encouraging to read during that dark time. This book is about detoxing your faith by tackling the toxins that have polluted it, and I saw many people's faith get polluted after the church's death. So here I go. If you are a new friend, dear reader, just read between the lines, and if you are an old friend, well, you will be able to fill in the blanks, take a walk down memory lane and smile with me at the end.

Painting with a very, very (did I mention very?) large brush, here is the scene: Church launches. Hundreds come. Leadership grows. Lives are changed. Healings manifest. Prophecies flourish. Pastor evolves. Apostolic ties are cut. Accountability declines. Rumors fly. Eldership probes. Pastor resigns. Membership dwindles. Interim pastor arrives. Hope resurrects. Former pastor divides. Stumbles and falls. Rumors are confirmed. Attendance plummets. Finances nosedive. Staff leaves. Members mourn. Families scatter. Leadership clashes. Tempers flare. Estrangements are born. Doors close.

So that is the plight of our wonderful, ten-year, near-million-dollar ministry in 62 words. The enemy struck our shepherd and the sheep scattered, and no matter how gallant the efforts of the second shepherd were, it was a flock marked for slaughter (see Zechariah 11:4–17).

Maybe you have not experienced a church hit, but a church split. We attended a funeral once where we were unsure if the man was a Christian or not. At the service we learned that he was indeed a Christian, and that he had even taught Sunday school forty years prior. But when a church split caused him great anger, he vowed never again to enter the doors of a church. He kept that vow for forty years, probably until he was wheeled in for his funeral.

How very sad to let one person's or one group's transgressions decide your spiritual fate! It made me sad, although we were at least happy to know that he was a Christian; it provided us with more hope that he was now with God.

If your church has undergone a hit or a split, you know that it evokes emotions and summons responses in you that you probably did not even know existed. It is likely that you will see the best and worst of yourself. The strongest and weakest. Here is a survival checklist for you if you are currently in this set of circumstances.

1. Get wise counsel, preferably from whoever oversees your church's ministry.

2. Pray and fast. But, should things drag on, limit the number of forty-day fasts you will do. Desperation, stress, lack of rest and excessive fasting caused me to throw my metabolism out of whack. God knows your heart. You do not have to kill yourself to keep your church alive.

3. Guard your tongue. Do not gossip. *Under. Any. Circumstances.* Trust me, the grace will be there for you to give people facts without being divisive. You can have opinions without being opinionated. You can judge without being judgmental.

4. If you are a leader, meet with members who might have questions and help bring them comfort. No gag orders. Information ends speculation and breeds peace and hope. Encourage people to stick it out and pray.

5. Watch at least two funny movies a week. I am serious. Laughter is good medicine! Remember that in ten years this will all be a dim memory, and new ones will have replaced it.

I am very sympathetic to church dramas and traumas. I know what it is like to have your church's survival be the last thing on your mind before you go to sleep and the first thing on your mind as you wake (and to dream about it all night long). There were nights that I had to sing my husband to sleep. We would often just rest and hold each other and let the tears come as we prayed. Little did we know that all those tears would water and grow a new church. We had no idea God was calling us to be pastors. We were so busy trying to love and mend people that it sort of sneaked up on us. We are still getting to love and mend new people today.

In retrospect, being in the marvelous ministries of those churches provided us with the opportunity to serve in and acquaint ourselves with every area of a church, which I think equipped us for where we are now: We have served in children's ministry, youth ministry, young marrieds and families, as deacon, as elder, as a prophetic voice and now as pastors. We love every inch of the Church. You will still find us mopping floors and taking out the trash. As I said, every inch.

Corresponding Emotional Toxins

People who have experienced a church hit or split often struggle with the emotions of abandonment, rejection, grief, anger and, eventually, isolation. Let's pray now for God to renew your mind and spirit from these potential influences and help your faith recover:

> *Father God, I know You love Your Bride more than I do. I know I am just a small part of Your Church, but God, I am hurting. I am angry at what has passed and fearful of what might come. I give You my rejection, grief and anger. Protect me from isolation due to abandonment. I will promote peace and devote myself to prayer. Give me favor with those whose ears You need me to fill with wise words. I rebuke the devourer from this ministry, and I shut the jaws of death that are causing gossip and speculation. May truth prevail. May love win. May peace come. In Jesus' name, Amen.*

Correlating Physical Detox

Today and tomorrow we cleanse the urinary system. Cranberries are known to have a powerful healing impact on the kidneys, so feel free to add a handful of fresh cranberries or straight cranberry juice—not juice cocktail—to your "Warrior Tonic."

Breakfast	The New Kidney on the Block Blast
Mid-a.m. Juicing	Warrior Tonic
Lunch	Pick Six Detox Soup
Snack	snack liberally from your yellows
Dinner	choose one green and one yellow fruit or vegetable (see Recipes for prep ideas); pair with brown rice or quinoa tossed with section spices and section nuts or beans
Nightcap	Detox Tea

Closing Blessing

May God heal your urinary system of any toxins and bless its cleansing as He heals your heart and faith of the toxins accumulated during any church trauma, drama or spiritual abuse.

DAY 6

Spiritual Toxin: Catastrophic World Events

You have heard it asked before: "Why does God allow natural disasters?" What they are really asking is, "Why does He allow bad things to happen to good people?"

The implication is that with all the terror going on in the world, God surely is not as powerful or compassionate as we claim He is, if He exists at all.

But you have to admit: The list is pretty imposing. When you try to wrap your head around the statistic of almost a quarter of a million people dying in 2004 from one earthquake, it is hard to comprehend. My son-in-law, Sgt. Kyle Caldwell, was a U.S. Marine corporal in the Indian Ocean headed toward Guam when that 9.3 earthquake gave birth to the world's most devastating tsunami. His ship was rerouted to Sri Lanka to help with the cleanup and humanitarian aid after the death and displacement of those many hundreds of thousands.

The Haitian earthquake of 2010, with its 52 aftershocks, killed even more than that—316,000—injuring another 300,000 and taking down 280,000 buildings. Or what about the East Pakistan (now Bangladesh) cyclone of 1970, which took half a million lives? Or the Shaanxi earthquake of 1556 in China, which killed 830,000? And speaking of China, what about the 1931 floods along the Yellow River, which were estimated to have killed between one and three million people via drowning, disease and resulting famine and drought? The same river had flooded fewer than fifty years before, killing just as many.

From the 2003 European heat wave that killed seventy thousand to the European Black Death—or Bubonic Plague—that killed almost seventy million in the mid-fourteenth century, Europe has seen her share of tragedy, too.

And then there are manmade calamities that need only one word or two to jar your memory: 9/11, Chernobyl, Exxon Valdez, *Challenger* explosion, the *Titanic*. The list goes on and on.

I think one of the hardest ones for me to swallow is when a statistic-worthy death toll is caused by injustice, as when the Nazis rose to power in 1933 in Germany, resulting in the extermination of more than six million Jews. The Holocaust. Or the Atlantic slave trade, which lasted from the fifteenth century until the nineteenth century, when it was finally abolished. American and European settlers captured and exploited West African men, women and children for plantation work, first subjecting them to unspeakable abuse during the voyage from Africa to the Americas (called the Middle Passage). It is imaginable that as many as sixty million Africans died or were enslaved as a result of these various slave trades.

And as if it is not bad enough that millions and even billions of lives have been lost in world disasters, there have been millions and billions of dollars lost, too. Chernobyl cost $200 billion alone.

And since we are discussing expensive world disasters, might I point out that the 2012 American presidential election saw more than $7 billion (yes, *billion*) spent in campaigning alone? As a result of the exorbitant cash flow, the Federal Election Commission processed eleven million pages of campaign-related documents in 2012. I am sorry, but that figure is only going to increase in future elections and *that* is definitely disastrous.

Although my research could not produce a total for all the monies spent on all the world's wars (and world wars) in history, surely, even without inflation allowances, the figure is in the quadrillions. The United States alone spends more on annual military defense than the next eleven countries combined—a staggering $577 billion a year. That is correct. We spend more than China, Russia, Saudi Arabia, the United Kingdom, Japan, Germany, France, India, Brazil, Italy and South Korea combined. According to Jorn Madslien, as reported by the BBC in 2009, "Indeed, some $2.4 trillion . . . or 4.4%, of the global economy 'is dependent on violence,' according to the Global Peace Index, referring to 'industries that create or manage violence'—or the defense industry."[2] In other words, war is big business.

In the worldwide cataclysms, wars and natural disasters, I wonder how many of the victims were children? Is not God the weatherman who could have prevented all those droughts, earthquakes, tsunamis, typhoons, cyclones, tornados, hurricanes, mudslides, wildfires and avalanches? I mean, think of it. Was God on vacation those days? What was He doing during Hurricanes Katrina and Andrew? Did He evacuate Louisiana as officials advised both times? Of course not.

When someone asks you why God allowed all of these disasters to occur, what do you say? What is your personal opinion on the matter? How would you explain it to a child?

We must gain a biblical perspective on catastrophic world events. Jesus said they would happen. Let's take a look at His words from Matthew 24:3–8 (NASB).

> As He was sitting on the Mount of Olives, the disciples came to Him privately, saying, "Tell us, when will these things happen, and what will be the sign of Your coming, and of the end of the age?" And Jesus answered and said to them, "See to it that no one misleads you. For many will come in My name, saying, 'I am the Christ,' and will mislead many. You will be hearing of wars and rumors of wars. See that you are not

frightened, for those things must take place, but that is not yet the end. For nation will rise against nation, and kingdom against kingdom, and in various places there will be famines and earthquakes. But all these things are merely the beginning of birth pangs."

We see in the book of Genesis that God designed the global laws of nature that still govern the earth today. The hard facts are that tornadoes are caused by unstable updrafts and downdrafts that interact with wind shears, and earthquakes are caused when rocks underground break along a fault line. So, we see that it is easy to see *how* natural disasters happen. What is not so easy to see is *why*.

We call them "acts of God," and yet I wonder: Does anyone also credit God with the centuries of peaceful seas and tranquil skies?

It must sadden God—who created the Garden of Eden to be a perfect place for humankind—to see what sin has done to His perfect world. Just as God permits wicked people to perform wicked acts, He also permits the earth to demonstrate the consequences that wickedness has had on His creation. Listen to Romans 8:20–21 (NLT): "Against its will, all creation was subjected to God's curse. But with eager hope, the creation looks forward to the day when it will join God's children in glorious freedom from death and decay."

While we must be cautious in our human assessment of natural and manmade disasters, not be judgmental and not claim that we know the reasons why God allows them, it is safe to say that each and every dark day on earth can be traced back to when darkness jealously invaded the earth through sin after God declared, "Let there be light." That is the answer we should give people when they ask why disaster comes. And to those in the midst of the disaster, we must respond with love and aid.

Corresponding Emotional Toxins

People who have lived through or been affected by natural or manmade disasters often struggle with the emotions of grief, doubt, anger and judgment. Let's pray now for God to renew your mind and spirit from these potential influences and help you recover:

Father God, it must be hard for You to watch Your perfect creation suffer the consequences of sin. So much unnecessary suffering. If only the whole world would turn to You! I pray it will. And I pray that in the meantime, the innocent who suffer grief, doubt, anger or judgment as a result of catastrophic events will be comforted and provided for. Use my hands to accomplish this. Guard me and mine with Your protection in these troubling times. In Jesus' name, Amen.

Correlating Physical Detox

Today we finish cleansing the urinary system. Repeat yesterday's meal plan, experimenting with this section's colors.

Closing Blessing

May God cleanse your entire urinary system and repair what needs healing as He cleanses and repairs your faith from any aftershocks of world catastrophic events.

SECTION **4**

Financial Toxins

Spiritual Emphasis: Receiving encouragement for disheartening financial frustrations, battles and setbacks. Learning how to walk in God's prosperity in all areas of life

Emotions Associated with These Toxins: frustration, jealousy, anger, rejection, stress, confusion, guilt, doubt, fear, defensiveness, apathy, failure, embarrassment, despair, shame, humiliation, disappointment, dissatisfaction, greed, lust, discouragement, weariness

Bodily Systems Detoxed:
Days 7 and 8: Endocrine (hypothalamus, pancreas, pituitary, thyroid, adrenals, pineal gland)
Days 9 and 10: Nervous (brain, spinal cord, nerves)
Days 11 and 12: Reproductive (ovaries, testes, hormones)

Section Colors

Besides the specified greens, this section's support colors are *white* and *tan*. These specific vegetables and fruits are colored by pigments called anthoxanthins, containing varying amounts of phytonutrients. This section's phytonutrients, such as allicin, sulphoraphane and quercetin, all help promote healthy cholesterol levels (which is a main ingredient in our most important hormones). The compounds in this section's white and tan colors bolster many parts of the body, including the endocrine system, the brain and hormones.

As a side note on phytonutrients, *phyto* refers to the Greek word for *plant*. Unlike the vitamins and minerals that plant foods contain, phytonutrients are not necessarily mandatory for keeping you alive, but when you eat or drink them, they keep your body working optimally and help fight disease. There are more than 25,000 phytonutrients found in our plant foods. Phytonutrients actually travel all the way to the cellular level deep into the genetics into a cell's nucleus, changing the very expression of your genes. This is very good news if one of your genes is beginning to express disease.

Section Grocery List

Purchase one or two of each of the following fruits and vegetables, depending on your appetite level. If the fruit or vegetable is tiny, purchase enough for at least two cups. In the case of leaf vegetables, one head, bunch or bag of each variety mentioned will suffice. You may also double up on one vegetable or fruit if you dislike another, but be open to trying new things! With each section you will better be able to gauge your appetite and adjust your purchases to accommodate it.

Whites/Tans	cauliflower, mushrooms, onions, parsnips, potatoes, white corn, Jerusalem artichokes, meat of banana, brown pear, apple, white nectarine
Greens	broccoli, spinach, asparagus, kale, turnip greens, romaine lettuce, avocado, kiwi
Allowed Additions	quinoa, brown rice; white beans, navy beans, flax seeds, brown eggs, grade B organic pure maple syrup, dark chocolate, coffee beans tossed sparingly into smoothies; oils: olive, coconut and/or flaxseed; chicken broth; once or twice a week you may trade your vegetable snack for a shake (see Recipes)
Herb/Spice Options	vanilla, nutmeg, cinnamon, garlic, ginseng, turmeric, rosemary, parsley
Tea	dandelion, milk thistle (see Recipes); options: echinacea, chamomile, passionflower; for flavor add an extra bag of any caffeine-free fruit or berry tea
Optional Meat	only vegetables are recommended, but a three-ounce serving of organic poultry or fish (size of deck of cards) is permitted at dinner
Nuts	pistachios, pecans, hazelnuts
Water	drink half your body weight in ounces daily
Bases for Smoothies	choice of milks: organic 2%, unsweetened almond, coconut; choice of waters: coconut or aloe
Rest	nine hours nightly

DAY 7

Spiritual Toxin: Lack of Promotion

I am one of those gals who do all their shopping online. I research, compare, read reviews and then make my final purchase choices. I will never forget the day, years ago as a new online shopper, when I noticed that tiny text field at checkout preceded by the phrase *enter promo code*. I quickly Googled it to see what it was and discovered a whole new world of price cuts and discounts. With little effort, too. You just Google the name of the online retailer, and you will find promotional codes, if they exist. It is as easy as copy, paste and save. For someone like me, that amounts to huge annual savings. Retailers do this because they know they can reach customers like me and stimulate sales through these types of promotions.

Would not it be wonderful if promotion in life worked the same way? Just enter a code and promotion comes your way? Well, what would you say if I told you that is how it works?

Let's look first at what the word *promotion* means. The term *promo* is a 1960s abbreviation of promotion. But the word *promotion* itself is a combination of late Middle English words: In Latin *promot* means "moved forward"; *promovere* comes from *pro* meaning "forward, onward" and *movere*, which means "to move."

So we see that the word *promotion* actually means "to move forward." Sort of the way a promotional code prompts you to move forward with an online sale. Except in real life, the forward motion affects whatever is at stake: your job, relationships, health, etc.

So have you ever felt as if your life is more anti-motion than pro-motion? Is there something you can do to get more substantial pro-motion? Let's see what God's Word says about it.

1. **Lest you be tempted to think that promotion comes from a boss, know that promotion actually comes only from God:** "For promotion and power come from nowhere on earth, but only from God. He promotes one and deposes another" (Psalm 75:6–7 TLB).

2. **Promotion comes when the favor of God comes:** "May the favor of the Lord our God rest on us; establish the work of our hands for us—yes, establish the work of our hands" (Psalm 90:17 NIV).

3. **We are to work unto God and not just for promotion by man:** "Whatever you do, work heartily, as for the Lord and

not for men, knowing that from the Lord you will receive the inheritance as your reward. You are serving the Lord Christ" (Colossians 3:23–24).

4. **Promotion comes after we humble ourselves:** "Humble yourselves before the Lord, and he will exalt you" (James 4:10).

5. **Promotion comes in God's timing:** "But as for me, I trust in You, O LORD, I say, 'You are my God.' My times are in Your hand" (Psalm 31:14–15 NASB).

6. **Wisdom will get you promoted:** "The wise are promoted to honor, but fools are promoted to shame!" (Proverbs 3:35 TLB).

7. **A lack of obedience can lift promotion from your life:** "So when Ahijah heard her at the door, he called out, 'Come in, wife of Jeroboam! Why are you pretending to be someone else?' Then he told her, 'I have sad news for you. Give your husband this message from the Lord God of Israel: "I promoted you from the ranks of the common people and made you king of Israel. I ripped the kingdom away from the family of David and gave it to you, but you have not obeyed my commandments as my servant David did. His heart's desire was always to obey me and to do whatever I wanted him to"'" (1 Kings 14:6–8 TLB).

8. **Good things come with true promotion:** "Then the king promoted Daniel and gave him many great gifts, and he made him ruler over the whole province of Babylon and chief prefect over all the wise men of Babylon" (Daniel 2:48 NASB).

9. **The promotion of good people means everybody benefits:** "When good people are promoted, everything is great, but

when the bad are in charge, watch out!" (Proverbs 28:12 MESSAGE).

10. **When the godly are promoted, God is promoted:** "Then Nebuchadnezzar said, 'Praise be to the God of Shadrach, Meshach and Abednego, who has sent his angel and rescued his servants! They trusted in him and defied the king's command and were willing to give up their lives rather than serve or worship any god except their own God. Therefore I decree that the people of any nation or language who say anything against the God of Shadrach, Meshach and Abednego be cut into pieces and their houses be turned into piles of rubble, for no other god can save in this way.' Then the king promoted Shadrach, Meshach and Abednego in the province of Babylon" (Daniel 3:28–30 NIV).

So to receive and understand promotion fully, we have to receive and understand those ten truths. I guess you could say that if there were a promo code for *promotion*, it would be this:

PROMO10

I leave you with this blessing from Psalm 20:4: "May he grant you your heart's desire and fulfill all your plans!"

Corresponding Emotional Toxins

People who feel that promotion constantly eludes them often experience frustration, jealousy, anger, rejection, stress and confusion. Let's pray now for God to renew your mind and spirit from these potential influences and to help you set new standards for yourself that will benefit your faith:

Father God, I acknowledge that promotion comes in Your timing and with Your favor, and I know that happens only when I am walking in humility and wisdom. I know that if I am not obedient, I am in danger of promotion passing me by. But I also know that when I am promoted, it will be for the good of all and that You will be promoted, too. God, I give You my future. Help me to wait on You and to resist frustration, jealousy, anger, rejection, stress and confusion. You will not forget me! I will work as unto You and expect to attract the attention of those around me for good, bringing glory to Your name. In Jesus' name, Amen.

Correlating Physical Detox

Today and tomorrow, we cleanse the endocrine system.

Breakfast	The Endocrine Energy Boost
Mid-a.m. Juicing	Laura's One-Two Punch
Lunch	Sixcess Salad
Snack	snack liberally from your whites/tans and greens
Dinner	choose one green and one white/tan fruit or vegetable (see Recipes for prep ideas); pair with brown rice or quinoa tossed with section spices and section nuts or beans
Nightcap	Detox Tea

Closing Blessing

May God regulate your endocrine system and your responses to financial stress as you wait for your season of promotion.

DAY 8

Spiritual Toxin: The "Sincome" Tax

You already know that it is possible to sin with your body. You know it is possible to sin with your words, thoughts and feelings. But did you know it is possible to sin with your finances? Oh, yes. Sin + Income = Sincome.

Listen, it is no secret that the last thing to get saved is a person's wallet. But part of seeking first the Kingdom is giving to God from your first fruits. It says, "I am Yours, God." It screams, "Everything I have is Yours." It proves to the enemy that you trust your Father. But how do you give to God? You cannot put your money into an envelope and mail it to heaven, right? So how do you accomplish giving to God? Let's look at what He Himself says.

> "Will a man rob God? Yet you have robbed Me! But you say, 'In what way have we robbed You?' In tithes and offerings. You are cursed with a curse, for you have robbed Me, even this whole nation. Bring all the tithes into the storehouse, that there may be food in My house, and try Me now in this," says the Lord of hosts, "if I will not open for you the windows of heaven and pour out for you such blessing that there will not be room enough to receive it."
>
> Malachi 3:8–10 NKJV

So this says plainly that if you do not tithe you are robbing God and are under a curse. But what is a "tithe"? It is the Hebrew word *maàser*, and means "a tenth; tenth part; tithe, payment of a tenth part." In fact, the GWT actually says, "Can a person cheat God? Yet, you are cheating me! But you ask, 'How are we cheating you?' When you don't bring *a tenth* of your income and other contributions" (emphasis added). There you go. Sincome.

Now that we have established what a *tithe* means, let's see what *storehouse* means, because that is where you are supposed to bring the tithe, and you need to be crystal clear where that is. It is the Hebrew word *'owstar* and means, among other things, "treasury." And "storehouse," of course. But God also says in the same verse (verse 10) "My house." This is the Hebrew word *bayith* and means "place, household, family, descendants as organized body, household affairs and receptacle." And what does *receptacle* mean? "Container, holder, repository, box, tin, bin, can, canister, case, bag." Sounds like an offering plate to me. And the "place, household, family and organized body" is the church. Your local church. Note that it also means "household affairs." This describes perfectly the business responsibilities of running a local church. It takes money to run a business or a household, and it takes money to run a church.

So now you know the "what" of tithing (to supply for God's work), the "where" of tithing (into the storehouse treasury, God's house, His local churches), the "why" of tithing (to give to God, not rob Him and receive provision), and the "how" of tithing (to give 10 percent of your income). That means one-tenth of your income each and every pay period, although I suppose you could bring it in lump sums at other times. That is not helpful, though, for assisting in the regular business transactions that every local church has. Keeping the lights on, paying for the facility, paying the staff who minister in the church all week long (or at allotted times) and, of course, serving the community and the world through missions. So it is best to carve the tenth off the top of your income each pay period. It is between you and God if you tithe from the gross or from the net.

The "tithe" is mentioned between thirty and forty times in Scripture, and it is called "holy to the Lord." Two of those passages are: "Every tithe of the land, whether of the seed of the land or of the fruit of the trees, is the LORD's; it is holy to the LORD" (Leviticus 27:30), and "You shall tithe all the yield of your seed that comes from the field year by year" (Deuteronomy 14:22).

And let me take a moment and address a controversial passage that many Christians quote in order to wiggle out of tithing. It is 2 Corinthians 9:7: "Each one must give as he has decided in his heart, not reluctantly or under compulsion, for God loves a cheerful giver."

Many believers quote this to say that the tithe, the tenth, is no longer required, but that each one must give whatever he decides himself and never out of "compulsion" (obligation or pressure). But that is the farthest thing from what this verse means! This is Paul taking up an offering for another group of Christians at another church who need help! It is basically a love offering or a missions offering. Look at 2 Corinthians 9 again, this time reading the six verses preceding verse 7 (this time in the NLT):

> I really don't need to write to you about this ministry of giving for the believers in Jerusalem. For I know how eager you are to help, and I have been boasting to the churches in Macedonia that you in Greece were ready to send an offering a year ago. In fact, it was your enthusiasm that stirred up many of the Macedonian believers to begin giving. But I am sending these brothers to be sure you really are ready, as I have been telling them, and that your money is all collected. I don't want to be wrong in my boasting about you. We would be embarrassed—not to mention your own embarrassment—if some Macedonian believers came with me and found that you weren't ready after all I had told them! So I thought I should send these brothers ahead of me to make sure the gift you promised is ready. But I want it to be a willing gift, not one given grudgingly. Remember this—a farmer who plants only a few seeds will get a small crop. But the one who plants generously will get a generous crop. You

must each decide in your heart how much to give. And don't give reluctantly or in response to pressure. "For God loves a person who gives cheerfully."

So here we have Paul in Macedonia writing to the church in Corinth about helping believers in Jerusalem. It is a missions collection or a love offering! Verse 2 even uses the word *offering*, so it is obviously not referring to their tithes. Paul is saying that with our offerings, we can give cheerfully whatever we purpose in our hearts and with no obligation. Just remember from our previous Malachi 3 study that tithes and offerings are different in God's definition. Thus, tithes are strictly defined as the tenth that you bring into God's house (His church) for household affairs, and offerings are whatever amount you want to give above that to whomever and wherever, cheerfully as you have purposed in your heart.

And lest this look as though I am promoting tithing because I am a pastor who wants to pad my wallet with my congregants' hard-earned money, let me remind you that Chris and I receive only a small stipend each for our work at Eastgate. There have been times, in fact, when we have given up our paycheck entirely when the church needed it. We do not pad our wallets, Chris and I. In fact, we love to see our congregants' wallets padded and blessed by God—the biblical way—becoming Kingdom funders. It was Martin Luther who said, "There are three conversions a person needs to experience: The conversion of the head, the conversion of the heart and the conversion of the pocketbook." I am happy to say we see all three at Eastgate Creative Christian Fellowship.

Personally I think the tithe should apply to every piece of income that comes into your household. This means from bonuses, royalty checks, garage sales and lemonade stands. You might find that extreme, but Chris and I have seen God bless it again and again. Tithing blesses the family wallet and has the ability to heal an overburdened one by lifting a curse from it. Remember the promise at the end of Malachi: "'Try Me now in this,' says the LORD of hosts, 'If I will not open for you the windows of heaven and pour out for you such blessing that there will not be room enough to receive it.'"

Corresponding Emotional Toxins

Christians who do not tithe often experience emotions of guilt, doubt, fear, apathy and defensiveness. Let's pray now for God to renew your mind and spirit from these potential influences and to help you set new standards for yourself that will benefit your faith:

> *Lord, I give You my finances; 100 percent of it came from You and is Yours. I ask You to increase my faith to tithe regularly (or to keep tithing), and ask You to smile upon my giving and bless it. I trust You. I cannot "outgive" You. Forgive me for any time I have entertained doubt, fear, apathy or defensiveness concerning tithing, and take my guilt. In Jesus' name, Amen.*

Correlating Physical Detox

Today, we finish cleansing your endocrine system. Repeat yesterday's meal plan, experimenting with this section's colors.

Closing Blessing

May God daily resource the needs of your hypothalamus, pancreas, pituitary, thyroid, adrenals, pineal gland and hormones, and may you increase your faith to resource the needs of His church with your tithes and offerings.

DAY 9

Spiritual Toxin: Can't Seem to Get Ahead

Boy, oh, boy. What a grim star-studded lineup so far in this section's topics on finances! We have dealt with your job ("Lack of Promotion") and your paycheck ("The 'Sincome' Tax"); and today's "devo" (devotional) addresses a financial "feeling." A despair among people who feel unable to get ahead. Sometimes in life you just feel stuck. There are many popular lists out there that tell you how to get ahead in life. There are many Christian lists out there about how to get blessed and stay blessed. I want to offer you a list of a different kind. A "backwards" list. This list is going to tell you what *not* to do if you want to stay stuck and never live up to your financial potential. You ready?

1. Do not tithe.

(Please see "The 'Sincome' Tax.") Some say that tithing is Old Covenant (Old Testament) and that we, as Christians, are not under that any longer. Yet they live their lives by the Ten Commandments and other Old Testament truths and promises, so that is a double standard. It is not up for debate that we should live our lives by the Ten Commandments, and it is not up for debate that we should tithe. Besides, tithing is in the New Testament, too. Of the thirty to forty times tithing is mentioned in Scripture total, three to four of those are in the New Testament. (I find it interesting that a "tithe" of all the tithe Scriptures are in the New Testament.) Malachi 3 states clearly that if we do not tithe we are robbing God and are under a curse. So my number-one suggestion for you if you do not want to get ahead in your finances, relationships, career, ministry or be blessed at all—and really want to stay stuck where you are and live under a curse—is never to tithe.

2. Do not give.

Again, "giving" is different from "tithing." When churches take up "tithes and offerings," the tithe is the minimum (the tenth of your income), and an offering is anything above that. God mentions in the Malachi passage we studied that you rob Him by not giving tithes *and* offerings, so those can definitely be brought into the church too, although later in the verse it only says, "bring all the tithes into the storehouse." So you can also give your offerings to others. Coats for the poor, donations for charities, etc. Those things are beautiful offerings, but your tithe is never to be used for them. "Tithes *and* offerings" clearly indicates that they are separate.

3. Be ungrateful.

I told a couple of my adult kids about this "backwards" list and asked them to contribute. Jude, my twenty-year-old, said quickly, "Be ungrateful." I have always taught my kids that ingratitude is a sin, and I see it is paying off. You do not want to fall into Paul's list from 2 Timothy 3:1–2 (NLT): "In the last days there will be very difficult times. For people will love only themselves and their money. They will be boastful and proud, scoffing at God, disobedient to their parents, *and ungrateful*" (emphasis added).

4. Be undisciplined.

Being undisciplined and lazy will take you where you want to go, *if* where you want to go involves poverty and lack. The Bible actually labels a person like this: "sluggard." Proverbs 20:4 says, "The sluggard does not plow in the autumn; he will seek at harvest and have nothing." And Proverbs 26:15 (NIV) says, "A sluggard buries his hand in the dish; he is too lazy to bring it back to his mouth." If you do not want to get ahead in life, be an undisciplined sluggard.

5. Complain a lot.

This one is contributed by my 23-year-old daughter, Jeorgi, who interestingly enough is *not* a complainer. Have you ever known one? *To complain* means to "grumble, bellyache or gripe," and as pastors we see our fair share of people who have not yet made the connection between their griping and their lack of progress. Do not forget Paul's words in 1 Corinthians 10:10 (ISV) about what God thought of the murmuring Israelites: "You must stop complaining, as some of them were doing, and were annihilated by the destroyer." So, friend, if you want your hard work constantly to be destroyed, complain.

6. Be disorganized.

We already mentioned lazy sluggards, who are usually very disorganized, but even the brightest and hardest working people can be disorganized, so this is not a problem limited to personality. Through organization, you will be able to set a budget, keep up with what gets spent where—and let's not forget ordering your schedule so that after you work hard, you have time to play and rest equally as hard. Jesus is our greatest example of an organizer: "And when it comes to the church, he organizes and holds it together, like a head does a body" Colossians 1:17 (MESSAGE). If you want to stay "stuck" where you are, be disorganized.

7. Think you are self-made.

Be proud and brag. This is another one from Mr. Jude, and perhaps you have known people like this before. They give no credit to God for the forward progress in their careers, ministries, families or finances. These are the good ole' boys (or gals) who tell you that hard work is the only thing that will get you anywhere—and they leave faith and God totally out of the mix. If you want to bring your successes to a crashing halt, tell Him you achieved them all yourself.

8. Do not take faith-risks.

Progress involves risk. Not irresponsibility, but risk. It is taking a chance and putting it all on the line (not to be confused with gambling). When you have a word from God about following Him to unknown territory—emotionally, geographically or occupationally—and it is backed up by wise counsel and God's perfect timing, great things can happen. ". . . Barnabas and Paul, men who have risked their lives for the name of our Lord Jesus Christ" (Acts 15:25–26). If you never want to go to a new level in your life, do not take faith-risks.

9. Settle for less.

Another one from Miss Jeorgi, and a good one. What are your expectations from God? Do you long for anything better than you have right now? Not because you are dissatisfied or greedy, but because you are His child and deserve His best? When is the last time you asked God for something that only He can accomplish for you? "You do not have because you do not ask" (James 4:2 NKJV). If you never want to get ahead in life, settle for less.

10. Be impatient.

So if you will just do steps 1–9 (or *not* do them, actually) and apply all of those ingredients to your living and giving, the last ingredient is just to be patient and let it all "bake." Cookies removed too soon from the oven come out gooey, and plans removed from patience do not come out at all. If you do not want to succeed in life, be impatient. Or you can remember Psalm 27:14 and prosper! "Wait for the LORD; be strong, and let your heart take courage; wait for the LORD!" I have found that "stuck" is a false feeling. "In him we live and *move* and have our being" (Acts 17:28 emphasis added). So get moving!

Corresponding Emotional Toxins

People who feel "stuck" or sense a lack of momentum toward their future often struggle with feelings of failure, embarrassment, jealousy, despair and anger. Let's pray now for God to renew your mind and spirit from these potential influences and to help you set new standards for yourself that will benefit your faith:

Lord, I want to be "unstuck." I want to go somewhere new! I receive what You have for me. All of it! Heal me of the feelings of failure, embarrassment, jealousy, despair and anger I sometimes battle. You are my Provider! You have established specific plans to use and prosper me! I trust You to take me somewhere, God. Here we go! In Jesus' name, Amen.

Correlating Physical Detox

Today and tomorrow we cleanse the nervous system.

Breakfast	Brain Boosting Banana Choco Chip Smoothie
Mid-a.m. Juicing	Four-of-a-Kind
Lunch	Take-Five Stir Fry
Snack	snack liberally from your whites/tans and greens
Dinner	choose one green and one white/tan fruit or vegetable (see Recipes for prep ideas); pair with brown rice or quinoa tossed with section spices and section nuts or beans
Nightcap	Detox Tea

115

Closing Blessing

May God heal any infirmities or irregularities in your brain as He simultaneously reinforces or rewires your thinking about tithing, giving, being disciplined, ceasing from complaining, getting organized, staying humble, taking faith-risks, never settling for less and finally, being patient for God's blessings to manifest.

DAY 10

Spiritual Toxin: Homeless or Houseless

Jesus said, "I go to prepare a place for you" (John 14:2).

First, a question: Do you have your own home?

Well, as of 2012, America had 86,985,872 homeowners, a number that represents approximately 65 percent of the United States' housing market. According to the U.S. Census Bureau, *homeowner* is defined as "an owner-occupied house" and not necessarily as a unit owned without a mortgage or debt. This figure dipped after World War II but has remained consistent since the 1960s.

Evidently, 81 percent of married couples own their own homes, while that number drops to between 47 percent and 58 percent for singles. Age plays a role, as well: 81 percent of all homeowners are over age 65, but under the age of 35, that number falls to 37 percent. Geographics are a factor, too, because the chances are higher that you own your own home if you live in eastern or central portions of America rather than in the West. For example, 75 percent of West Virginians and Michiganians own their own homes versus only 55 percent of Californians.

While those are great figures for the American economy, more than thirty countries hold higher home ownership statistics than the United States. Romania is at the top with 97 percent, Lithuania 92 percent, Singapore and Hungary 91 percent, China and Slovakia 90 percent, India 87 percent, Mexico and Italy 80 percent, and Canada 69 percent. South Korea, Germany and Switzerland have some of the world's lowest home ownership rates at 54, 53 and 44 percent respectively. Where do you fall within those statistics?[1]

I ask because there is a prevalent opinion in the world that you are not successful until you own your own home. Again, I am not speaking of owning the title, but at least of having a mortgage. Somehow, this is synonymous with affluence, even though that affluence comes at a high price. Americans are notorious for assuming irresponsible amounts of debt; but, of course, nobody has to know that and *will not* know that as long as the landscaping outside of said house and the shiny new car in the driveway of said house are equally as perfect as it is. International economies would recover overnight if the world would just obey the Tenth Commandment: "You shall not covet your neighbor's house; you shall not covet your neighbor's wife, or his male servant, or his female servant, or his ox, or his donkey, or anything that is your neighbor's" (Exodus 20:17).

But even with that truth in mind and with all the international statistics laid out for you to see, I want to encourage you today if you are someone who wants to buy your own home and never seems to be able to, or perhaps you do have a mortgage and you long to pay it off. Either way, please know that the desire to have your own place comes from above and is God-inspired. Even the nation of Israel cried out to God because they desired a home of their own, and they got one.

So, then, if having a home to call your own is a God-given desire, why does it seem hard to achieve sometimes? Simply put, I believe the enemy desires God's children to be homeless. After all, he and his spirits are homeless, too, and always searching for someplace or someone to occupy. They are jealous of having a peaceful residence, so they do whatever they can to prevent it for everyone else, especially for believers. This includes influencing you with temptations to misspend your money and become poor and financially unstable with bad credit so that you cannot afford your own home. So stay smart—and stay encouraged—that God is on your side for you to have your own place to call home, and that all you need do is obey and honor Him with your income, saving, spending and tithing.

I have known adults who had to go back home to live with parents for a season. Or with siblings or friends. With several children in tow! I myself had to move back in with my mother and step-dad once while we were waiting for the closing of our first home. What was supposed to be a few days turned into about six weeks, and I had a husband and our first baby! My mom worked it out for her company's distribution truck to hold all of our belongings from our little apartment, and it sat in the company parking lot for weeks just waiting for the closing date. It was not easy, but I was so, so grateful to Mama and David for working it all out for us. God bless you if you have ever received anyone into your home for a season. It is a sacrifice of love!

But if you are one of the 35 percent of Americans (or 3 percent of Romanians, etc.) who do not currently own their own homes due to some extenuating circumstances—voluntary or involuntary—take heart! If it is a desire of yours to have your own "home sweet home," keep trusting God and stewarding your finances. The day will come when you will be the one opening your doors for others in need.

We stayed in that first little house for almost five years and have now lived in our current house for more than 25 years. It is known as "Campsmith," and, oh, if these colorful walls could speak! Six children were raised here (four born while here), eight grandbabies have come across the threshold, and let's not forget all the bustling birthday, anniversary and holiday parties, countless bridal and baby showers, incalculable church meetings and counseling sessions and prayer gatherings, numberless written and recorded songs, at least a dozen books and possibly hundreds of scripts, an infinite number of videos edited, untold handcrafted wood projects and room remodels, and, of course, twenty-plus rewarding years of homeschooling. Surely the Creator dwells here with all that creativity oozing from the woodworks.

But we almost lost this precious house three times in about a seven-year span when we were living by faith and in training for ministry. During those hard years, we (Chris, our six kids and I) all worked together to meet the monthly mortgage and to keep the lights on. It is hard for parents to need help from their children, but our family has always been a team, and so we exhibited the finest teamwork anywhere during those years. Chris and I were working hard to make ends meet, and yet there were months when the kids had to pitch in with their babysitting money, lawn-mowing funds or money earned from a local talent agency that had gotten them involved in doing commercials, music videos and more.

Chris and I kept a spreadsheet of what we owed each child and paid them back once we got back up on our feet, but all we could corporately think of at the time was to save "Campsmith" (which evidently is a person, place or thing). I am so thankful to God for those people who sowed into our family during those years, too, and how thankful I am still sitting here in this house, writing yet another book.

May God give you your own camp, too, or bless the one you already have. Then you can say what we say about Campsmith: "This is God's camp!" (Genesis 32:2).

Corresponding Emotional Toxins

People who feel homeless in one way or another often struggle with feelings of shame, jealousy, despair and humiliation. Let's pray now for God to renew your mind and spirit from these potential influences and to help you set new standards for yourself that will benefit your faith:

Lord, I want to be a good steward of all You have given me and will continue to give to me. I want to use my home to be a blessing to all who know me, and so I ask You to make a way for that to happen. I declare that no matter where I dwell, You will dwell there with me. In Jesus' name, Amen.

Correlating Physical Detox

Today we finish detoxifying the nervous system. Repeat yesterday's meal plan, experimenting with this section's colors.

Closing Blessing

May God heal any issues in your central nervous system, which is the body's headquarters for all its various operations, and may He establish you in your own home, which is your own personal headquarters, refuge and sanctuary.

DAY 11

Spiritual Toxin: "Stuffopedia" (The Debtor's Diary)

I do not like to shop. I like to buy. To me, the endless searching, walking and price foraging is a waste of precious time. If I had my way, I would know precisely what I want, the exact store it is in, the exact aisle it is on, and then I would whisk in, pay and whisk right back out. As I said in "Lack of Promotion," I do most of my shopping online.

If you are like that, too, then, evidently, you and I are a minority. In a 2013 article in the business section of *The Atlantic* entitled, "Wanting Expensive Things Makes Us So Much Happier Than Buying Them," it is proposed that more pleasure is often achieved from the wanting than from the owning. In other words, unlike me, most people like to shop. In fact, they love the pursuit of the item so much that the purchase is often followed by a letdown. "Materialists are more likely to overspend and have credit problems, possibly because they believe that acquisitions will increase their happiness and change their lives in meaningful ways," Marsha L. Richins of the University of Missouri concludes in her paper "When Wanting Is Better Than Having."

But in three separate studies, materialists reported significantly more happiness thinking about their purchases beforehand than they did from actually owning the things they wanted. "Thinking about acquisition provides momentary happiness boosts to materialistic people, and because they tend to think about acquisition a lot, such thoughts have the potential to provide frequent mood boosts," Richins says, "but the positive emotions associated with acquisition are short-lived. Although materialists still experience positive emotions after making a purchase, these emotions are less intense than before they actually acquire a product."[2]

Look around your house right now, or at what you are wearing. Can you remember when and where you bought the shirt you have on? What about some of the objects to your left or right? What about the shoes on your feet or the flooring under them? Do you remember the rush and joy of these purchases?

I buy very deliberately. When there were eight people living in our home before any of the children moved out, we had little room, so nothing was brought home unless we knew where it would go and what purpose it would serve (even if it was just for pleasure). I learned to purchase intentionally and never impulsively. When I worked as a TV host on the Shop At Home Network, we knew how to compel impulse buyers into a purchase. Impulse buyers were those who could be spontaneously motivated to buy. I would not call it manipulation—it was not like we were ringing up purchases on their credit cards without their permission—but we definitely knew how to get them to pick up their phones. I sometimes wonder where all of those products are that I sold to people. They were quality products, so I hope they are still enjoying them! But at the end of the day, it was all just "stuff."

If we all are not careful, we can fall into the stuff pit. Admit it: You like your stuff! But purchasing stuff without restraint can leave you with a false sense of self, not to mention in serious debt. Consider these questions:

- *If every debt you owed was paid off and you had no payments, what could you live on?*

- *If you cut out the majority of your coffee runs and meals out, how much would you save monthly? What would you put that money toward?*

- *What items do you have right now that you can sell and start paying off some debt?*

- *Do you have two of some items? Three? And why? If there is no good reason, which one of those duplicates can you sell or gift?*

"Don't store up treasures here on earth, where moths eat them and rust destroys them, and where thieves break in and steal" (Matthew 6:19 NLT).

I remember one fiscally challenging year I had four yard sales within eighteen months. We needed the funds and my closets and cabinets needed purging, so I was fine with the extreme stuff liquidation. I did the fourth sale because we desperately needed new kitchen flooring. By faith, I got the estimate, which was $337.00. Then I planned the sale, wondering what on earth I had left to offer since all the other sales had really gotten rid of all our excess. But we needed that flooring, so I dug deeply in every drawer and under every bed.

We did well, but by the end of the second day I was still $36.30 short, and I was determined to raise all the monies with my garage sale. At the last minute, a woman drove up and saw a wall plate set I owned. I had saved those expensive plates for twenty years because you are supposed to hang on to collector's items, right? But this particular set was worth more than a hundred dollars, and I doubted the woman was going to pay that much at a garage sale.

When she approached me with the set to inquire, I hesitated as I thought about their worth. But then, I realized at that moment that those plates were just stuff. Did I want those plates hidden in a closet or did I want new flooring for all to see? When the woman asked me how low I would go on the plates I blurted out, "$36.30!" She probably thought I had lost my mind, but she gladly dug the money from her purse and took her plates. She got a deal and I got my flooring. What a feeling! Maybe you should consider your goals or needs and have your own "extreme stuff liquidation."

Another stuff-liquidation method I use is participating in online trading posts. There is usually one in every community on Facebook. One Christmas, I sold enough of my excess stuff to buy a new iPad for my husband and a new iPhone for my son, with cash. My husband and I always discuss major purchases together, and so you should have seen his face when he opened his brand-new $500 iPad. I said, "Not to worry, I merely sold the baskets, books, those extra comforters, etc. . . . ." It is amazing how all your accumulated stuff adds up. These online forums are great because you do not have to lug your belongings out into the yard and weather the elements. Just snap a pic, upload and wait for the offers. Both of these stuff-liquidation ideas—coupled with exercising restraint when making new purchases—will keep you from falling into the stuff pit.

We have all heard of those hoarding shows, and if you have not watched one you need to, especially if you have issues with stuff. It is time for you to clean out, donate, give or sell. And if you do not have an immediate goal that you need the funds for, consider putting that money away for a rainy day. We all know that they come.

One last assignment for you: Go find a picture of yourself from twenty years ago or more, one in which you are in a room in your own home, or what was your home if you are in a different one now. Next, look at every item in that photo around you. All the stuff. Chances are that you do not even own any of it anymore. I did this recently with a picture of me in my first home holding my daughter Jessica. I had tediously decorated that room, and if I close my eyes I can remember the saving, fretting, swatching, shopping and returning that went into the total "experience" of that room. But as I looked at this picture recently, I realized that the only thing I still owned from that photo was . . . my daughter. It put all my stuff into perspective.

There is nothing wrong with liking your stuff. I even love some of my stuff. I just think that most of us need to redefine "enough."

Corresponding Emotional Toxins

People who spend excessively, accumulate unhealthy debt, hoard their "stuff" or need material things to stay happy often experience emotions of disappointment, dissatisfaction, greed, lust and jealousy. Let's pray now for God to renew your mind and spirit from these potential influences and to help you set new standards for yourself that will benefit your faith:

> *God, I am sorry for any time I have overemphasized material things, and I ask You to reset my spending priorities. Show me whom I need to share my possessions with, or what I can liquidate to reduce my debt. I surrender to You my occasional feelings of disappointment, dissatisfaction, greed, lust and jealousy. I declare that I will live a debt-free life, live within my means and trust You to be the sole source of my happiness! In Jesus' name, Amen.*

Correlating Physical Detox

Today and tomorrow we cleanse your reproductive system.

Breakfast	The Hormone Fixer Elixir
Mid-a.m. Juicing	Warrior Tonic
Lunch	Pick Six Detox Soup
Snack	snack liberally from your whites/tans and greens
Dinner	choose one green and one white/tan fruit or vegetable (see Recipes for prep ideas); pair with brown rice or quinoa tossed with section spices and section nuts or beans
Nightcap	Detox Tea

Closing Blessing

May God heal your reproductive system of any infirmity, including infertility, hormonal imbalances, prostate issues and more, and may you contemplate what might be limiting your productivity in life, including the way you handle your personal finances or spending that might be preventing God's blessings from flowing freely toward you.

DAY 12

Spiritual Toxin: Get Rich Quick (Losing the Lack Mentality)

We have spent a lot of time admonishing and challenging during this section, so I want to make sure that you are encouraged with the understanding of this vital truth: *God wants you to prosper.* If I can convince you of that before we leave here, then you are wealthy already. I call that revelation, "Getting Rich Quick."

Those words—*God wants to prosper you*—summon different convictions and even prejudices in different camps. So now, those of you who do not believe that God wants to prosper His kids are expecting me to end this devotional by saying that all the anti-prosperity folks out there need to accept the fact that God wants us all to drive Cadillacs, own massive homes and live lavish lives. Those of you who do believe in "the prosperity message" are expecting me to end this devotional with the predictable reminder that true prosperity includes being wealthy in family, peace and health. Well, I am not going to go the predictable route, but I do think both camps are going to be pleased with where this devo lands.

First, did you know that the Bible mentions money more than 2,300 times? It is, in fact, the most-mentioned topic in Scripture. Twice more than heaven and hell combined, thrice more than love, seven times more than prayer and eight times more than belief? Depending on the translation you use, the word *give* appears 921 times in Scripture, almost as many times as *love* (541), *faith* (270) and *hope* (165), added together.

Perhaps this shows that giving *is* an expression of faith, hope and love. But the topics of money, possessions, generosity, treasures, giving and related issues are the focus of seventeen of Jesus' 38 parables (that is almost half), and comprise 15 percent of God's total Word. This information was gathered by the National Christian Foundation (the Indiana branch), which is the twelfth largest charity in the nation and deals entirely with educating Christians in wise money management so that we might be able to resource the advancement of God's Kingdom. They believe there is a "modern day generosity movement" in which God is moving hearts to give as never before, but that it all begins with solid biblical training regarding personal money and finances.[3]

There is no denying that there is a primal connection between our spiritual lives and how we handle money. Jesus even said, "For where your treasure is, there your heart will be also" (Matthew 6:21). If you want to learn a lot about a person, take a look at two things—his checkbook and his calendar—and you will see where his priorities lie. So is it any wonder that the Bible gives so much attention to the heart-revealing topic of money?

I want to allow God's Word to speak for itself to you about your money, including God's desire to prosper you, but also to help you to learn to give, save, budget and more. Out of the more than 2,300 Scriptures on money, I have compiled my personal top twenty and put them into ten practical categories that I believe God wants you to be convinced of and live by. So grab a cup of tea and let these powerful Scriptures make you rich, "quick."

God wants you to give.

The righteous gives and does not hold back.

Proverbs 21:26

"Give, and it shall be given unto you; good measure, pressed down, and shaken together, and running over, shall men give into your bosom. For with the same measurement that ye mete withal it shall be measured to you again."

Luke 6:38 KJV

God wants you to be compassionate to the poor.

He who gives to the poor will never want. But he who shuts his eyes will have many curses.

Proverbs 28:27 NASB

He who is generous will be blessed, for he gives some of his food to the poor.

Proverbs 22:9 NASB

God wants you to love Him and not money.

"No one can serve two masters, for either he will hate the one and love the other, or he will be devoted to one and despise the other. You cannot serve God and money."

Matthew 6:24 NET

"You shall generously give to him, and your heart shall not be grieved when you give to him, because for this thing the LORD your God will bless you in all your work and in all your undertakings."

Deuteronomy 15:10 NASB

God wants you to prosper.

Beloved, I wish above all things that thou mayest prosper and be in health, even as thy soul prospereth.

3 John 2 KJV

He will be like a tree planted by the streams of water, that brings forth its fruit in its season, whose leaf also does not wither. Whatever he does shall prosper.

Psalm 1:3 WEB

God wants you to receive.

Furthermore, as for every man to whom God has given riches and wealth, He has also empowered him to eat from them and to receive his reward and rejoice in his labor; this is the gift of God.

Ecclesiastes 5:19 NASB

The blessing of the LORD makes a person rich, and he adds no sorrow with it.

Proverbs 10:22 NLT

God wants to provide for you.

"Do not worry then, saying, 'What will we eat?' or 'What will we drink?' or 'What will we wear for clothing?' For the Gentiles eagerly seek all these things; for your heavenly Father knows that you need all these things."

Matthew 6:31–32 NASB

And Abraham calleth the name of that place "Jehovah-Jireh," because it is said this day in the mount, "Jehovah doth provide."

Genesis 22:14 YLT

God wants you to learn to save and budget.

"Four things on earth are small, yet they are extremely wise: Ants are creatures of little strength, yet they store up their food in the summer."

Proverbs 30:24–25 NIV

Good planning and hard work lead to prosperity, but hasty shortcuts lead to poverty.

Proverbs 21:5 NLT

God wants you to be content.

The LORD is my shepherd, I shall not want.

Psalm 23:1 KJV

Keep your life free from love of money, and be content with what you have.

Hebrews 13:5

God wants you to be out of debt.

Evil men borrow, but do not repay their debt.

Psalm 37:21 NET

Better not to vow than to vow and not pay.

Ecclesiastes 5:5 NKJV

God wants you to understand that prosperity is conditional.

"Submit to God and be at peace with him; in this way prosperity will come to you."

Job 22:21 NIV

And keep the charge of the LORD your God, to walk in his ways, to keep his statutes, and his commandments, and his judgments, and his testimonies, as it is written in the law of Moses, that you may prosper in all that you do, and wherever you turn yourself.

1 Kings 2:3 AKJV

I hope that these verses will transform your financial future. I hope that no matter which "camp" you considered yourself in at the start of this devotional, you will now see that the "prosperity gospel" that I believe in is a conditional, hardworking, big-vision, money-making, Kingdom-funding, pleasure-bringing, God-glorifying gospel! I hope you agree. When Paul said in 1 Timothy 6:10 (KJV), "For the love of money is the root of all evil," please note that he did not say money is evil. He said the *love* of money is the root of all evil. So I close this section on financial toxins by reminding you to love God—never your money—and to manage your character and your money as if they decide your net worth together, because they do. Remember: "A good name is more desirable than great riches" (Proverbs 22:1 NIV).

Corresponding Emotional Toxins

People who do not know that God wants to prosper them often experience emotions like doubt, fear, discouragement and weariness. Let's pray now for God to renew your mind and spirit from these potential influences and to help you set new standards for yourself that will benefit your faith:

> *Lord, it is consistent with Your character as a loving Father that You want to bless and prosper me. I am sorry for entertaining emotions like doubt, fear, discouragement and weariness. I trust Your many thoughts toward me! Help me to be compassionate to the poor, put You first above money, believe You want me to prosper, receive Your provision, learn to save and budget, be content and live debt-free. I know that prosperity is conditional. I pray I will make wise choices that attract Your blessings. In Jesus' name, Amen.*

Correlating Physical Detox

Today we finish cleansing the reproductive system. Repeat yesterday's meal plan, experimenting with this section's colors.

Closing Blessing

May God balance your hormones so that your body operates to its fullest potential, and may God's provision and your stewardship of it help you yourself operate to your fullest potential in life.

SECTION **5**

Health-Related Toxins

Spiritual Emphasis: Acknowledging the faith-stealing questions we have about healing in Scripture, filtering past hurts over any unanswered prayers for healing, and building a strong biblical foundation for divine health so we can be more immune to bodily warfare

Emotions Associated with These Toxins: shame, jealousy, despair and humiliation, confusion, jealousy, doubt, pride, hopelessness, unhappiness, stress, distress, doubt, uncertainty, anger, weariness, disappointment, frustration

Bodily Systems Detoxed:
   Days 13 and 14: Respiratory (nose, lungs, pharynx, larynx, trachea, bronchi, alveoli)
   Days 15 and 16: Immune (bone marrow, thymus, glands)
   Days 17 and 18: Lymphatic (spleen, lymph nodes, ducts, tonsils)

Section Colors

Besides the specified greens, this section's support color is *purple*. These specific vegetables and fruits are colored by phenolic flavonoids called anthocyanins, which are water-soluble pigments that may appear purple or blue depending on the pH level. They contain anti-inflammatory, antiviral and anticancer benefits for the whole body, but there are specific foods within this color group that are especially beneficial for the immune, lymphatic and respiratory systems.

Cruciferous vegetables with these pigments, such as purple cauliflower, purple cabbage, purple kale and purple broccoli, have been shown to stop the progression of lung cancer and cut the risk in half of developing it to begin with, so we see they are advantageous to the immune system. But they are also good for the lymphatic system, as evidenced by the fact that their anthocyanin-rich nutrients and extracts have long been used to treat even the common cold.

As for the respiratory system, grape clusters uniquely resemble the alveoli of the lungs, so it seems almost providential that they have so many respiratory benefits, including reducing your risk of lung cancer and emphysema. Resveratrol is an antioxidant found in all grapes, but in larger quantities in purple and red ones (especially in the grape skins). Thanks to resveratrol, grapes can reduce inflammation-causing compounds on the lung's cell lining. As for grape seeds, they diminish the severity of allergy-induced asthma due to the chemical proanthocyanidin. Pomegranate juice, which also contains these purple-hued pigments with powerful antioxidants, has also been found to slow the growth of lung tumors.

The lymphatic and immune systems are closely linked and their roles and parts overlap, but for this cleanse we have designated their components and organs as listed.

Section Grocery List

Purchase one or two of each of the following fruits and vegetables, depending on your appetite level. If the fruit or vegetable is tiny, purchase enough for at least two cups. In the case of leaf vegetables, one head, bunch or bag of each variety mentioned will suffice. You may also double up on one vegetable or fruit if you dislike another, but be open to trying new things! With each section you will better be able to gauge your appetite and adjust your purchases to accommodate it.

Purples	purple onion, purple carrot, purple potato, purple cauliflower, purple cabbage, purple bell peppers, purple asparagus, eggplant, plums, prunes, elderberries, purple (or red) grapes, blueberries, blackberries, pomegranate
Greens	green bell peppers, Brussels sprouts, celery, spinach, kale, pear, kiwi, cucumber, broccoli, limes, kelp, capers, avocado, endive, parsnip
Allowed Additions	quinoa, brown rice; banana, pinto beans, lima beans, cranberries and raw cranberry juice; oils: olive, coconut and/or flaxseed; chicken broth; once or twice a week you may trade your veggie snack for a shake (see Recipes)
Herb/Spice Options	cinnamon, garlic, oregano, parsley, cilantro, mint leaves, thyme, eucalyptus, sage, rosemary
Tea	dandelion, milk thistle, echinacea; booster option: decaf green tea; for flavor add an extra bag of any caffeine-free fruit or berry tea
Optional Meat	only vegetables are recommended, but a three-ounce serving of organic poultry or fish (size of deck of cards) is permitted at dinner
Nuts	Brazil nuts, almonds, cashews
Water	drink half your body weight in ounces daily
Bases for Smoothies	choice of milks: organic 2%, unsweetened almond or coconut milk; choice of waters: coconut or aloe
Rest	nine hours nightly

DAY 13

Spiritual Toxin: The Cure for Sick and Tired (The Ten Healing Commandments)

Have you ever been sick? Yes. Have you ever been tired? Yes. But they are two totally different conditions than "sick and tired"!

"Sick and tired" implies a span of time. A drawn-out battle with no end in sight. And whether or not the battle originated in your body, it eventually finds its way there.

Well, God does not want us to be sick, tired or "sick and tired," and if you are any of those three today, I have good news for you!

In this section of the book we will explore the faith toxins that infect your views on healing inch by inch. God wants you well! Some of you might not have known that God still heals, but He does, and the only way to be convinced of that is by showing you His Word. It is what convinced me!

When I began discovering healing Scriptures for the first time, however, I became overwhelmed. Not only because I was ashamed of not knowing how many there were from Genesis to Revelation, but also because I did not know where to begin to learn to "pray" them. Counting all the Scriptures, stories, miracles and testimonies about healing, miracles or the faith required for them, there must be more than a thousand biblical references. I wanted to memorize them all! I knew according to Ephesians 6 that the Word of God is our sword, but I felt as if I had been handed one thousand swords and did not know which one to pick up first. I wanted to wield them all with strength. Taking into account that Hebrews 4:12 says the Word of God is a double-edged sword, that is a lot of sharp metal to wield.

But practice makes perfect. Over the last twenty-plus years I have honed my sword-fighting skills by discovering which of my healing swords produce what result. For example, when you are sick as a result of your own doing (bad food choices, wounds after a fight, etc.), you need Psalm 103:2–3: "Bless the Lord, O my soul, and forget not all his benefits, who forgives all your iniquity, who heals all your diseases." But when you get a fatal diagnosis from a doctor, you need Jeremiah 30:12, 17: "For thus says the Lord: Your hurt is incurable, and your wound is grievous. . . . For I will restore health to you, and your wounds I will heal, declares the Lord."

For this very reason, I created The Ten Healing Commandments. It does not categorize healing Scriptures so much as it trains you how to posture yourself for healing. It was my cure for "sick and tired," and it can be yours, too. Are you ready? Commit them to memory:

1. I am the Lord, your Healer, and thou shalt have no other healers before Me.

> "For I am the Lord, your healer."
>
> Exodus 15:26

2. Thou shalt receive My healing Scriptures.

> He sent out his word and healed them, and delivered them from their destruction.
>
> Psalm 107:20

3. Thou shalt not be offended at healings or miracles.

> "The blind receive their sight and the lame walk, lepers are cleansed and the deaf hear, and the dead are raised up, and the poor have good news preached to them. And blessed is the one who is not offended by me."
>
> Matthew 11:5–6 (see Luke 7:22)

4. Thou shalt live righteously in gratitude for My Son's stripes.

Who his own self bare our sins in his own body on the tree, that we, being dead to sins, should live unto righteousness: by whose stripes ye were healed.

1 Peter 2:24 KJV

5. Thou shalt not fear sickness.

"For thus says the LORD: 'Your affliction is incurable, your wound is severe. There is no one to plead your cause, that you may be bound up; you have no healing medicines. . . . I will restore health to you and heal you of your wounds,' says the Lord."

Jeremiah 30:12–13, 17 NKJV

6. Thou shalt take care of your body.

Do you not know that you are God's temple and that God's Spirit dwells in you?

1 Corinthians 3:16

7. Thou shalt eat your fruits and vegetables.

And God said, "Behold, I have given you every plant yielding seed that is on the face of all the earth, and every tree with seed in its fruit. You shall have them for food."

Genesis 1:29

8. Thou shalt ask for the anointing oil.

Is anyone among you sick? Let him call for the elders of the church, and let them pray over him, anointing him with oil in the name of the Lord. And the prayer of faith will save the one who is sick, and the Lord will raise him up. And if he has committed sins, he will be forgiven.

James 5:14–15

9. Thou shalt believe.

And he did not do many mighty works there, because of their unbelief.

Matthew 13:58

10. Thou shalt lay hands on the sick.

"And these signs will accompany those who believe: in my name they will cast out demons; they will speak in new tongues; they will pick up serpents with their hands; and if they drink any deadly poison, it will not hurt them; they will lay their hands on the sick, and they will recover."

Mark 16:17–18

I encourage you to memorize these Ten Healing Commandments and then heed them. When you are sick, when you are tired, and especially when you are sick and tired of being sick and tired.

Corresponding Emotional Toxins

People who are "sick and tired" due to battling health issues often struggle with feelings of weariness, discouragement, doubt and hopelessness. Those who do not understand God's healing promises can often experience offense over them. Let's pray now for God to renew your spirit and mind from these potential influences and to help you set new standards for yourself that will benefit your faith:

God, You are my Healer. I surrender to You my spirit, soul and body, and ask You to invigorate all three. I receive Your healing Scriptures, will not be offended at Your miracles, am grateful for Jesus' stripes, and will not fear sickness. I vow to You to take care of my body by eating the vegetables and fruits that fight illness, and by asking for the anointing oil and the prayer of faith when illness fights back hard. I will fight unbelief and choose faith, and I will impart that to others when I lay hands on the sick. I give you my weariness, discouragement, doubt, hopelessness and any offenses. I trade them today for healing. In Jesus' name, Amen.

Correlating Physical Detox

Today and tomorrow we cleanse the respiratory system.

Breakfast	Love Your Lungs Smoothie
Mid-a.m. Juicing	Laura's One-Two Punch
Lunch	Sixcess Salad
Snack	snack liberally from your purples and greens
Dinner	choose one green and one purple fruit or vegetable (see Recipes for prep ideas); pair with brown rice or quinoa tossed with section spices and section nuts or beans
Nightcap	Detox Tea

Closing Blessing

May God cleanse your respiratory system and fill your lungs with new breath and your mouth with praise so that you are no longer sick and tired (spirit, soul or body).

DAY 14

Spiritual Toxin: When Healing Will Not Come

I remember when I first started to believe in divine healing based on God's Word. After 25 years of being in church (since infancy) and 15 years of that spent being a Christian, Scriptures were suddenly illuminated to me that I had missed after all those years of reading, learning and teaching the Bible. This coincided with increasing health concerns that left me desperate for healing, and over the course of the next three very strategic years, God grew me in faith and convinced me unequivocally that He could and *would* heal me.

I tell the entire story in chapter 9 of *Seeing the Voice of God: What God Is Telling You Through Dreams and Visions*, and I urge you to read it in full, because many have told me they relate to the progressive healing journey I have had. Even if healing had not been promised in God's Word to me, I also had dramatic encounters and visitations during that time in which God told me forthrightly He would heal me. But in one dramatic visitation on January 26, 1994, God said He had already begun to heal me but that it would be "by process." It has indeed been a twenty-year-plus process now of gradual improvement. On a scale of one to ten, with ten being healed and one being the horrible neurological condition I once lived in, I would say I am now about a nine. I feel better than ever before in my life at age fifty, and through it all I have become a stronger, smarter and more disciplined woman of faith.

But along the way, the hardest part of the waiting was, surprisingly, not the physical symptoms that were in my body, but the psychological warfare in my mind. The enemy's voice telling me God had not promised me healing. That I had misinterpreted the Bible. That I would never be well. What was equally as discouraging was when that discouraging voice came

141

out of mouths that I loved. It would set me back weeks. But eventually it was only days, and then hours, then minutes, then seconds and now, I can honestly tell you that I do not bat an eye at the enemy's discouragements. No matter if they come from Satan—the father of lies himself—or from someone who does not realize he is using them to discourage me. Besides, people have marked my progress and seen what God has done for me, and so now all the naysayers are gone! Vanished!

But of utmost importance to my faith was an enlightening, overlooked scriptural truth I discovered unexpectedly. While chatting with the Lord very casually about something totally unrelated, my mind—without my help—suddenly began reflecting on a list of the nine spiritual gifts of 1 Corinthians 12. I knew this was the Lord's influence. Suddenly, I saw something I had missed. First, here is the subtext verse: "A spiritual gift is given to each of us so we can help each other" (1 Corinthians 12:7 NLT), and then come the gifts:

1. word of wisdom
2. word of knowledge
3. faith
4. gifts of healing
5. the working of miracles
6. prophecy
7. discerning of spirit
8. speaking in tongues
9. interpretation of tongues

What I noticed was found in gifts 4 and 5. Healing and miracles. I had always regarded them as the same. But I saw that if God had outlined nine distinct gifts in this passage, then surely all nine were different. If healing and miracles were the same, then why were there not only eight gifts of the Spirit? Then I saw in verse 28 that God distinguished them again: "And God has appointed in the church first apostles, second prophets, third teachers, then miracles, then gifts of healing, helping, administrating, and various kinds of tongues."

There He went again, segregating miracles and healings! I set out to discover why. Let's first look at two of the New Testament Greek words for *miracle. Dynamis*: "strength power, force, might, energy, physical power." And I love this particular definition, "the abstract for the concrete," because it indicates making something materialize from nothing, which would indeed be miraculous. It also means: "inherent power, power residing in a thing by virtue of its nature, or which a person or thing exerts and puts forth, the power for performing miracles, power consisting in or resting upon armies, forces, hosts." It is where our word *dynamite* originates. So we see that this is a "power" word.

Another Greek word for *miracle* is *semeion*. It means "a sign; a mark; a token; unusual occurrence, transcending the common course of nature; of signs portending remarkable events soon to happen; miracles and wonders by which God authenticates the men sent by him, or by which men prove that the cause they are pleading is God's." In other words, a sign to support the person preaching the Gospel at that moment so that all will know God is in their midst. So we see this is a "now" word.

Put together, these New Testament definitions of *miracle* seem to convey, "Power, now!" Next, let's look at the word *healing*, for it, too, has several New Testament Greek representations. See if you notice how these differ from the previous "power-now" word:

> *therapeuo* or *therapeia*: "a service rendered, specifically a medical service." (From where *therapy* originates.) So we see this is a "process" word.

143

kalos: "to be well and recover." We see this in Mark 16:18: "They will lay their hands on the sick, and they will *recover.*" Recovery, too, is a "process" word.

lama: "medicine; remedy; a means of healing." From *laomai*, meaning: "to cure or heal." Yet another "process" word. Medicine, remedies and cures take time.

So have you noted the difference yet between *miracle* and *healing*? A miracle is an instantaneous phenomenon, and a healing is a progressive phenomenon. Is either any less phenomenal? No! But one happens gradually, by process.

So perhaps you have prayed for a miracle, but instead you got only a healing. Wait . . . *only a healing?* Do you see the wrong mentality there? There is no shame in waiting on God! All that means is that He is requiring you also to focus on your spirit and mind being made whole, whereas with a bodily miracle you are not required to go deeper with the Lord and heal the other two-thirds of your person. Healings are an invitation. "Walk with Me. Trust Me. Recover with Me. Let *Me* be your therapy and cure." Healings bring wholeness, and wholeness is a process.

So if God were to produce an infomercial for miracles and healing, miracles would be the catch-your-attention product, but healings would be the "But wait! There's more!"

And those Greek and Hebrew words just scratch the surface in giving us insight. In the Bible, when you see the word *healing*, it could be one of fourteen Hebrew words or nine Greek words. They each hold keys for understanding the marvelous gift of wellness. Healings are not second-class answers to prayer. It just means you are in the middle of a miracle, so to speak.

In light of this study, do you now see the beauty in why God distinguishes these two spiritual gifts in 1 Corinthians 12? By doing so He is saying, "To some I have given the ability to work miracles, and to others I have given the ability to invent cures and medicines."

So when you pray for a miracle in your body, and you do not see it happen instantly, praise God out loud and tell all your friends, "I got my healing!" That is not just religious rhetoric. It means you are in process and on a beautiful journey with God toward wholeness, body, soul and spirit.

Corresponding Emotional Toxins

People who feel that wellness eludes them or who confuse healings with miracles often battle the emotions of confusion, jealousy and weariness. Let's pray now for God to renew your mind and spirit from these potential influences and to help you set new standards for yourself that will benefit your faith:

> *Lord, I see it in Your Holy Scriptures that You want me to be healthy. I invite Your health into my spirit, my mind and my body. I ask You for a miracle, Lord, but should You choose to do a work of wholeness in me and walk me through a process of recovery instead, then I submit to You. I resist the enemy's thievery, in Jesus' name, as well as the emotions of confusion, jealousy and weariness. By Your stripes, I am healed. In Jesus' name, Amen.*

Correlating Physical Detox

Today we finish cleansing the respiratory system. Repeat yesterday's meal plan, experimenting with this section's colors.

Closing Blessing

May God cleanse your respiratory system as you take a deep breath and take back your total temple health.

DAY 15

Spiritual Toxin: Thorns in the Flesh (Paul's Thorn, Part 1)

Today, I confront, head on, the passage that was always used to show me God did not want some people healed: the "thorn in the flesh" message in 2 Corinthians 12.

> So to keep me from becoming conceited because of the surpassing greatness of the revelations, a thorn was given me in the flesh, a messenger of Satan to harass me, to keep me from becoming conceited. Three times I pleaded with the Lord about this, that it should leave me.
>
> verses 7–8

Many, many Christians—after reading inaccurate commentaries or hearing flawed teachings by admired pastors—have interpreted it like this:

> So in order to keep me from being conceited, God gave me a disease or affliction, inspired by Satan, to torment me. Three times I begged God to take the disease from me and He refused, telling me grace was enough and that He wanted me to stay sick.
>
> 2 Corinthians 12:7–8, MCT
> (which is the Misled Christian's Translation!)

How preposterous! I have extensively studied this passage over the decades and have come to believe that Paul's thorn has nothing at all to do with a chronic sickness. Trust me, because of my bodily sufferings it would have been easier to believe it does! But I decided a long time ago to preach God's Word and not my experience. God's Word never changes, but my experience can and *will* if submitted to the totality of God's Word.

So it is going to take us a few days' worth of devo faith detoxes to unravel this highly disputed topic, but we must.

You see, Paul's thorn of the flesh has become a thorn in the flesh of Jesus' Bride, and I believe God wants it extracted from her once and for all. Why on earth would He go to so much trouble to remove every spot and wrinkle from her gown and not remove the thorn that could tear it to shreds? Let's get to work.

Whether you are trying to solve an actual crime or just playing the game of "Clue," you need to know three concrete things when solving a mystery: (1) the what, (2) the where and (3) the who ("Miss Scarlet, in the library with a candlestick!"). I am going to add the not-so-concrete why (the motive) since Paul's text includes one, too. So let's look at the clues in Paul's now-famous text, because by defining them we can unravel the thorny mystery. Today we tackle the first two:

1. The thorn (what)
2. Paul's flesh (where)

The thorn is the "what." It is the Greek *skolops* meaning "a stake" or "a thorn." It is used only once in Scripture. We know that Paul's thorn was metaphorical and not a literal thorn, or he would have used *akantha*, the word employed when describing Jesus' crown of thorns. Some have tried to make this metaphor a chronic sickness but none has stood the test of time. One such theory was that Paul's thorn was epilepsy; in fact, in Old Ireland, epilepsy was known as St. Paul's Disease. And many of those who support this theory point to Paul's Acts 9:3–9 Damascus Road blindness, not as an actual sudden vision loss but as the result of a hypothetical convulsion. In 1987, *The Journal of Neurology, Neurosurgery, and Psychiatry* published an article by D. Landsborough, which proposed that Paul's conversion experience, with the bright light, loss of normal bodily posture, a message of strong religious urging and his subsequent blindness, all evidenced "an attack of [temporal lobe epilepsy], perhaps ending in a convulsion. . . . The blindness which followed may have been post-ictal" (which is the period of groggy recovery immediately following a seizure).[1] But, thankfully, this Damascus Road seizure theory is refuted in the same journal by other scholars who say it does not account for Paul's companions hearing the voice (Acts 9:7), seeing a light (Acts 22:9) and falling to the ground (Acts 26:14). There is also no other place in all of Paul's letters (books) in which this very transparent author ever mentions having epilepsy. I have written many books and can tell you that all my previous seizure sagas (and triumphs through them) found their way into almost every one!

Bottom line is that Paul's thorn is not literal. It is metaphorical *about* something literal. If I, in a detailed, ten-page, six-thousand-word letter, mention to a friend, "I am 'sick and tired,'" will those who read it a hundred years from now think I was literally sick? And literally tired? Will they even understand I was just emotionally weary? They will if they read the rest of my long letter. So let's look at the rest of this portion of Paul's 6,239-word letter to the Greeks.

The "where" is Paul's flesh. First, we must consider some modern opinions about Paul's choice phrase "in my flesh." *Flesh* is the Greek *sarx* and means everything from "the soft substance of the living body, which covers the bones and is permeated with blood of both man and beasts" to "mere human nature, the earthly nature of man apart from divine influence, and therefore prone to sin and opposed to God." So this can be a body *or* mind word. Those who believe this *stake* was a bodily disease claim *sarx* as a body word and argue for a sensory defect, pointing to evidence of vision impairment through Paul's failure to recognize the High Priest (Acts 23:1–5), his large handwriting (Galatians 6:11) and the Galatians' willingness to have plucked out their eyes and given them to Paul (Galatians 4:15). But others—myself included—believe Paul used *sarx* as a mind word, referring to his "human nature, the early nature of man apart from divine influence." So when he said *skolops sarx* (translated as "a thorn in my flesh") he was using a metaphorical term to describe an inner struggle. For those who still think Paul had an eye disease, pointing to Galatians 4:15, where he references the Galatian people being willing to pluck out their eyes for him, let's back up two verses and go to the Greek. Galatians 4:13 (KJV) says, "You know how through weakness of the flesh I preached the gospel unto you at the first."

Weakness is the Greek *astheneia* and means "want of strength, weakness, infirmity; of the body, its native weakness and frailty, feebleness of health or sickness." Some translations used the word *illness* in place of "weakness," and yet nowhere is that found in the original Greek. The word also means "of the soul; want of strength and capacity; to bear trials and troubles." Once again, this can be a body *or* mind word. Combined, this suggests someone who is weak in body and mind, and therefore points directly to a gruesome stoning Paul had just received. Basically, in Galatians 4 he is referencing the stoning that occurred to him in Acts 14:19–20 just before he came to Galatia. The stoning wounded him so badly that he was presumed dead, but then verse 20 says the disciples stood round him and he rose up, departing with Barnabas to Derbe.

Well, scholars throughout the ages agree that the Galatian churches were in south Galatia and that a traveler would have had to pass through the Cicilian Gates and Derbe to get there. Thus, my hypothesis is that Paul arrived in Galatia weak in body and mind after a horrific stoning, needing recovery, and this was the *astheneia* weakness he referred to in Galatians 4:13, and possibly even the need for a new set of eyes in verse 15! It also convincingly accounts for the scars Paul mentions later in

Galatians 6:17: "From now on let no one cause me trouble, for I bear on my body the marks of Jesus."

But do you see, this was not a chronic (ongoing) illness? For someone to believe this Galatians 4:13 passage was an eye ailment, he or she must first be predisposed to the wrong thinking that Paul had a chronic disease, which unfortunately many point to 2 Corinthians' thorn reference to substantiate. But notice again the previously quoted Galatians 4:13 where Paul says his infirmity was "at the first," indicating it was not a permanent ailment at all but something temporary (like wounds from a stoning) that had now healed.

So if this thorn in the flesh is not a chronic disease, what was it and why did Paul choose this idiom? Well, what most people do not realize is that the scriptural idiom "thorn in my flesh" or "thorn in my side" did not originate with Paul, and that we see it first in the Old Testament.

Moses said in Numbers 33:55 (KJV): "But if ye will not drive out the inhabitants of the land from before you; then it shall come to pass, that those which ye let remain of them shall be *pricks in your eyes, and thorns in your sides,* and shall vex you in the land wherein ye dwell" (emphasis added). Judges 2:3 (KJV) says: "Wherefore I also said, I will not drive them out from before you; but they shall be as *thorns in your sides,* and their gods shall be a snare unto you" (emphasis added).

Joshua 23:13 (KJV) says: "Know for a certainty that the LORD your God will no more drive out any of these nations from before you; but they shall be snares and traps unto you, and scourges in your sides, and *thorns in your eyes,* until ye perish from off this good land which the LORD your God hath given you" (emphasis added). Does God's Word say that Moses, Samuel, Joshua and all of Israel were going to have literal thorns in their eyes or sides? No, and neither does it say that about Paul. Paul would have known about this scriptural phraseology and drawn from it.

Tomorrow we tackle what this inconvenient affliction was for Paul. I will give you Scriptures and you will have a choice to make. But for today, open your heart to the idea that God did not have plans for Paul to stay sick, nor does He have them for you.

Corresponding Emotional Toxins

People who misinterpret Paul's thorn passage (of which I was one) are often victims of bad teaching and struggle with confusion, doubt and pride (if they are refusing to consider a new interpretation). Let's pray now for God to renew your spirit and mind from these potential influences and to help you set new standards for yourself that will benefit your faith:

> *Lord, I seek truth. Correctly interpreting Paul's thorn passage is crucial for Your Church because its misinterpretation possesses the power to undermine the very work of the cross. Give me a mind to understand and discern, and I release to You any confusion, doubt or pride that I have accumulated over time concerning this passage. In Jesus' name, Amen.*

Correlating Physical Detox

Today we focus specifically on the immune system.

Breakfast	Lick the Spoon Immune Purple Slurp
Mid-a.m. Juicing	Four-of-a-Kind Juice
Lunch	Take-Five Stir Fry
Snack	snack liberally from your purples and greens

Dinner	choose one green and one purple fruit or vegetable (see Recipes for prep ideas); pair with brown rice or quinoa tossed with section spices and section nuts or beans
Nightcap	Detox Tea

Closing Blessing

May God cleanse your immune system as you ask Him to cleanse your mind from all wrong interpretations of Paul's thorn in the flesh.

DAY 16

Spiritual Toxin: Afflictions Working for You (Paul's Thorn, Part 2)

Earlier in Paul's second letter to the Corinthians, before all this "thorn" talk, he told them, "For our light affliction, which is but for a moment, works for us a far more exceeding and eternal weight of glory" (4:17 AKJV). So we see that our afflictions are working for us. Think of them as temporary employees hired to do a job, dismissed once their purpose is served. But who hires them? God? Satan? You? And why would God allow this hiring if it leads to your suffering? More on suffering tomorrow, but for today, we must first dig deeper into Paul's thorn because it holds a key for you. Here is 2 Corinthians 12:7–8 again:

> So to keep me from becoming conceited because of the surpassing greatness of the revelations, a thorn was given me in the flesh, a messenger of Satan to harass me, to keep me from becoming conceited. Three times I pleaded with the Lord about this, that it should leave me.

152

Yesterday we examined the "what" and the "where" of Paul's flesh thorn, and today, we turn our attention to the "who" and the "why." Who do you think gave Paul this thorn in his flesh, this "stake" in his "body and soul"? Was it God? Or Satan? Determining this will help us answer the "why," which is the motive of the giver.

1. A messenger (who)
2. The motive (why)

The "who" is a messenger of Satan. Looking at the 2 Corinthians 12:7 text, this one is pretty straightforward and simple. The thorn in the flesh is said to be "a messenger of Satan." *Messenger* is the Greek word *aggelos* and means "a messenger, envoy, one who is sent, an angel, a messenger from God." It appears 186 times in the New Testament. In 179 of these citations, it is translated "angel." In 7, it is "messenger." It is never expressed as anything else. When looking at all 186 of these usages, there is not one example contextually where it can be anything other than a living, feeling being. So there you have it: Paul's thorn in the flesh was not a "what" at all (including a sickness), but a "who"!

But you ask, "If that Greek definition is correct, how can 'a messenger from God' be an evil source of distress?" Well, remember that the fullness of that definition also includes "messenger, one who is sent, an angel," and so, since the actual Bible text reads, "a messenger [*aggelos*] of Satan," we see clearly that this must have been a dark angel, "a messenger of Satan sent to torment." In fact, the Weymouth New Testament translation of verse 8 says: "As for this, three times have I besought the Lord to rid me of *him*" (emphasis added). Not "it." "Him." But the flip side of this "who" is . . . who did the sending? God or Satan himself? The text does *not* say that Satan sent the messenger. It begins with, "I was *given*," which is the Greek *didōmi* and among other things means "to give over to one's care, entrust, commit." So this demon was sent by someone and given over to Paul. Entrusted to him. But who? We find the answer in the "why."

The "why" is the motive. I realize there are several of my fellow charismatic Bible teachers who believe Satan was behind the sending of this messenger, but there is a compelling argument for why I believe that God gave ("entrusted") the messenger of Satan to Paul. First, the opening words of the 2 Corinthians 12:7 text reveal the motive of the giver: "to keep me from becoming conceited." So, I ask you, would Satan really want to keep Paul's pride in check? Would the devil want to keep Paul from sinning? No. So we see that God is the mastermind behind this plan. He gave "it," and Paul knew it, because God is the one Paul went to thrice to ask for it to be taken away. Paul's heavenly revelations were so magnificent that the thorn (the messenger) was going to keep Paul humble, and, boy, did it work, because Paul was full of humility!

But the second reason this God-giver theory makes sense is because the Greek *didōmi* ("give") word reveals that God "entrusted" this dark angel to Paul. Why? For Paul to have authority (and to grow in his understanding of his authority) over the dark messenger. This entity had no authority over Paul, for the Lord would never allow a satanic being to have authority over one of His kids. God knew the future and already knew Paul would not become prideful. Remember, too, that God did not allow Satan to test Job to keep him from sinning, but to prove to Satan that he would *not* sin (and Job did not). Same here with Paul. I am convinced that God allowed this messenger to torment Paul, but that in the end, God's plan was for him to learn that this dark angel—and others like him—-were under his authority. In fact, this *didōmi* word is the same exact "give" word used in these other Bible passages about God giving Christians authority over demons:

Behold, I give [*didōmi*] unto you power to tread on serpents and scorpions, and over all the power of the enemy: and nothing shall by any means hurt you.

Luke 10:19 KJV

And when he had called unto him his twelve disciples, he gave [*didōmi*] them power against unclean spirits, to cast them out, and to heal all manner of sickness and all manner of disease.

Matthew 10:1 KJV

And I will give [*didōmi*] unto thee the keys of the kingdom of heaven: and whatsoever thou shalt bind on earth shall be bound in heaven: and whatsoever thou shalt loose on earth shall be loosed in heaven.

Matthew 16:19 KJV

So God "gave and entrusted" (*didōmi*) this dark messenger to Paul. It served a purpose in Paul's ministry. But what did this messenger actually do to make Paul's life so hard at times? Paul already told us in verses 9–10 of the 2 Corinthians 12 (KJV) passage:

Most gladly therefore will I rather glory in my infirmities, that the power of Christ may rest upon me. Therefore I take pleasure in infirmities, in reproaches, in necessities, in persecutions, in distresses for Christ's sake: for when I am weak, then am I strong.

Paul uses the word *infirmities* here, so some cite this as proof that he was describing a chronic disease. But the Greek word is *astheneia* (which we learned yesterday), and means "want of strength, weakness, infirmity; of the body, its native weakness and frailty, feebleness of health or sickness." It also means "of the soul; want of strength and capacity; to bear trials and troubles." Combined, this implies someone weak in body and mind (soul). True, the definition offers the options of "sickness" and "weakness,"

155

but I imagine that Paul's stonings, fastings and nakedness in the cold did make him weak and sick (not to mention seasick), yes? This is further proven in chapter 11 where he details his infirmities (*astheneia*), none of which is a chronic illness:

> Three times I was beaten with rods, once I was pelted with stones, three times I was shipwrecked, I spent a night and a day in the open sea, I have been constantly on the move. I have been in danger from rivers, in danger from bandits, in danger from my fellow Jews, in danger from Gentiles; in danger in the city, in danger in the country, in danger at sea; and in danger from false believers. I have labored and toiled and have often gone without sleep; I have known hunger and thirst and have often gone without food; I have been cold and naked. Besides everything else, I face daily the pressure of my concern for all the churches. Who is weak, and I do not feel weak?
>
> 2 Corinthians 11:25–29 NIV

Paul's infirmities (*astheneia*) were the dangers and persecutions he suffered because of the Gospel! Besides, he said earlier he would boast in his "infirmities"—plural—and so if you are going to claim Paul had a chronic disease you are going to have to claim he had several. More examples of these *astheneia* persecutions are given in Acts 9:23, 26–29; 13:6–12, 44–50; 14:1–19; 16:12–40; 17:1–14; 18:1–23; 19:23–31; and 20:3.

For those who still insist that these "infirmities" were chronic illnesses, it should be noted that every other major translation of the Bible chose the word *weaknesses* and not *infirmities*, including the NIV, NASB, NKJV, ESV, NLT, HCSB, ISV, NET, ASV, GWT, ERV, Darby translation and more. Paul's persecutions made him weak at times. Do yours? Of course.

So he was not allowed to boast about himself, but he *was* allowed to boast about his infirmities, which he outlined in detail in the many passages I just listed for you.

Christians have tried so hard over the years to stay sick. While in their hearts they would love to lay down their crutches, turn in their handicap signs and throw away their medicines, more often than not, when healing does not come they begin rearranging Scripture to fit their experience. I would think it would take less energy to accept the more than one thousand healing verses in Scripture than to go digging all over the Bible for proof that Paul was diseased. Why do we want to spend so much time proving God wants us to stay sick? Here is the reason: It helps us feel better when healing does not come quickly. It allows us to give up. The enemy smiles because he has convinced one more person not to fight him. And he did not have to do anything but whisper.

If we were in a court of law and God were on trial for failure to uphold His vow as Jehovah-Rapha ("the Lord who heals"), the judge would look at all the vast scriptural evidence of His Bible healings, allow testimonies of His continued healing power today and then look at this one, tiny passage about Paul's thorn and overrule its admission as legitimate evidence of misconduct, throw out the case, convict the plaintiff of perjury and declare God not-guilty. Case closed!

This tormentor was a thorn in Paul's side, but Paul was a thorn in "its" side too. Likewise, you can be a thorn in the side of any of Satan's messengers you encounter in life. Tomorrow we will learn how the thorn functioned in Paul's life and how he put the suffering to work for him. Remember, your afflictions are working for you!

Corresponding Emotional Toxins

People who live under constant affliction struggle with the emotions of hopelessness, unhappiness, stress and distress. Let's pray now for God to renew your mind and spirit from these potential influences and to help you set new standards for yourself that will benefit your faith:

Lord, I am no stranger to affliction, but neither were You. I see where Your afflictions were working for You, and I believe I can master and dismiss mine as well. I surrender to You any hopelessness, unhappiness, stress and distress I encounter. I call myself blessed. In Jesus' name, Amen.

Correlating Physical Detox

Today we finish cleansing the immune system. Repeat yesterday's meal plan, experimenting with this section's colors.

Closing Blessing

May God bless this detox and cleanse your immune system, which was designed to help your body fight off physical afflictions. Likewise, may God give you the keys to rid your life of the afflictions that torment you, putting them to work for you in the meantime.

DAY 17

Spiritual Toxin: Why Does God Allow Suffering? (Paul's Thorn, Part 3)

Maybe you are chronically sick in your body or love someone who is. Have you ever asked, "Why, God?" Have you ever dug into His Word and cried out for the answers to your suffering? If so, good for you, because so many people do not! They hear a well-meaning sermon that references Paul's thorn being a chronic disease, which he asked and was denied healing for three times, and walk away rationalizing that this is the explanation for why they were not healed. They asked, nothing changed, and so they assumed the answer was no. They skipped right past "wait and watch" or "learn to rebuke the enemy" or "have someone lay hands on you." Either that, or they heard the discouragingly interpreted thorn sermon and think, *Why bother asking for healing at all?* Or maybe they are just too lazy or busy to search it out for themselves in Scripture and learn the freeing truth. They have not because they ask not. So they stay sick.

But there is another group, one that is even more dangerous to the integrity of the full Gospel. It is those who hear this incorrect thorn theory and not only accept it, but wear it like a badge. Their badge says, "Leave me alone. God wills my disease." When I see, hear or discern this, it makes me grieve. It compromises the cross.

In this case, it is not God who is allowing their suffering, but themselves. Do they not see the countless Scriptures from Genesis to Revelation on divine healing? Many of them have. Then why do they not believe them? What has happened? It is obvious that two main toxins have infected their faith: (1) They or someone they love stayed sick or even died after they prayed for healing, and/or (2) they heard Paul's thorn message preached wrongly and embraced an incorrect teaching. This is why I deal with both of those topics in this book. I want to reach this crowd. I used to be among them.

Oh, how I wish I had never heard this incorrect teaching as a kid—from a pulpit, in a conversation, in a devotional—and had instead just found this passage myself without prejudice! From the text, it would not have entered my mind that God wanted Paul to suffer with a chronic disease! I would have interpreted it as it was intended—especially after studying the Greek meanings of the key words as we have here—and it would have saved me decades of suffering. But I did not know. I was lazy and did not study God's Word about healing. My suffering was not being allowed by God. It was being allowed by me.

Finally, in my late twenties, some sound teaching on Paul's thorn intersected with a sudden urgent need for me to be healed. I tell the full story in *Seeing the Voice of God*, but suffice it to say that I got desperate, and desperation is the cure for doubt and laziness. I was so relieved to learn that Paul's metaphorical phrase *thorn in his flesh; a messenger of Satan* was not an illness at all, but the weaknesses and persecutions brought on by being a follower of Jesus and promoting the Gospel. It changed the entire focus of my prayers, and catapulted me onto the healing path that has made me who I am. A healthier version than ever before!

But I sometimes wonder if Paul is in heaven watching billions of people read his thorn passage and thinking, *Why on earth did I choose those words? Why was I so metaphorical?* Goodness knows I have regretted an email or two. Or sometimes I wonder if the translators who chose the word *illness* are in heaven watching these thorny debates and second-guessing their interpretations. Probably not, and I am not suggesting erring on either's behalf! In fact, I think God may have left it somewhat ambiguous for a reason. Proof of this is that all the scholars who claim emphatically this is a physical illness cannot even agree on what it is. Epilepsy? Ophthalmic eye disease? Stuttering? Malaria? Leprosy? Depression? Headaches? Hysteria? Wow! Sounds crystal clear, right? To speculate is missing the point. The reason they cannot agree on an illness is because it *was not* an illness. Paul was not ill, he was under spiritual attack by a demonic antagonist. And it influenced as many people as it could to take him down. What the enemy did not anticipate is that while he was so busy persecuting Paul, a full documentation of Paul's victories over him were being recorded word by word, epistle by epistle, and now comprise more then two-thirds of the New Testament read by billions of believers on continents Paul never knew existed. Paul won by a landslide.

Paul listed his persecution "infirmities" multiple times in Scripture. And why did God deny Paul deliverance from them the three times he asked? Because God does not deliver us from persecution. Jesus told us it would come to us as it came to Him. And Paul reiterates this in 2 Timothy 3:12 (KJV): "Yea, and all that will live godly in Christ Jesus shall suffer persecution." *But*, God's grace is sufficient for us, just as it was sufficient for Paul. Just as it was for Jesus.

The truth is, if God stopped all persecution, Saul would have never become Paul. God allowed Stephen to be stoned to death, and Acts 7:58 says of the encounter: "Then they dragged him [Stephen] out of the city and began to stone him; and the witnesses laid their coats at the feet of a young man named Saul" (NRS). In chapter 8, Saul is still seen persecuting Christians, but at the start of chapter 9, Saul has his Damascus Road encounter and becomes Paul. The rest is history. But it all began with Stephen's persecution and stoning.

It is clear that the thorn in Paul's flesh was persecution. Persecution from the devil to prevent him from preaching the Gospel, and allowed by God to ensure he clung to it. Now *that* is what I call using what the enemy intended for evil for good!

Corresponding Emotional Toxins

People who question why God allows suffering sometimes wrestle with the emotions of doubt, uncertainty and anger. Let's pray now for God to renew your spirit and mind from these potential influences and to help you set new standards for yourself that will benefit your faith:

> *Father God, simply put, I hate suffering! I sometimes get angry when suffering comes because You are my father and I expect You to rescue me. Help me to see that You have already rescued me through Your finished work of the cross,*

and that it is up to me to enforce Your victory. You will not exempt me from persecutions any more than You did Your own Son, but You will train me to overcome them, one by one! This is the cure for my doubts and uncertainties, and for those of the people watching me. In Jesus' name, Amen.

Correlating Physical Detox

Today and tomorrow we focus specifically on the lymphatic system.

Breakfast	The Clean Spleen Cider
Mid-a.m. Juicing	Warrior Tonic
Lunch	Pick Six Detox Soup
Snack	snack liberally from your purples and greens
Dinner	choose one green and one purple fruit or vegetable (see Recipes for prep ideas); pair with brown rice or quinoa tossed with section spices and section nuts or beans
Nightcap	Detox Tea

Closing Blessing

May God strengthen your lymphatic system and bolster your faith as you seek Him concerning your sufferings.

DAY 18

Spiritual Toxin: The War on Wellness

This week we have talked about how God is our Healer of illnesses and our Deliverer from trouble, but not our preventer of persecution. Second Timothy 3:12 (KJV) says: "Yea, and all that will live godly in Christ Jesus shall suffer persecution," and sometimes that persecution comes in the form of attacks on our bodies (like Paul's many beatings, his stoning and other "*astheneia* infirmities"). As with Paul, God certainly has not spared me from the overall thorn of persecution, but He does teach me to war and allows me to partner with Him in prayer for my deliverance. In fact, He delivered me from one while writing these pages.

I was writing this section on health toxins during the week of my 31st wedding anniversary, and I took a two-day break so Chris and I could get away to our favorite bed-and-breakfast, Butterfly Meadows Inn and Farms in Franklin, Tennessee. Upon returning, I developed stabbing back pain, and by day two, I could not move. I could not stand without help or walk unassisted. I have never had back issues and was puzzled. In fact, the last time I had had a back injury was while writing *Seeing the Voice of God* when I had a freak fall, broke a back rib and punctured a lung, winding up on total bed rest. The majority of that book was written there! Well, here I was again. My bed had become my desk, and I could not even get up to eat with my family or to enjoy all my kids and grandkids who were gathering for Easter. The only thing that was pain free were my fingers, which thankfully was all I needed to keep writing, but when one of my fingers began to go numb, I realized what the enemy was up to. He was after my fingers, and so he struck my back so that a pinched nerve would numb and cripple my hands. He did not want me to write this book.

Then I had another revelation: This had something in common with the last time I was on bed rest, and it was not just that it was a back injury. It was that I was writing about the body and health both times. In *Seeing the Voice of God* there are two medical chapters that contain information on sleep cycles, an interview with a sleep study doctor, how to get better sleep and how to use nutrition to remember your dreams better. My injury happened while writing those health chapters, and now here I was again, writing to encourage people who need healing, with me myself laid up in a bed doing it. I. Got. Mad! Warfare prayer rose up within me, and I alerted my intercessory prayer team and asked them to let it rise up in them, too. The dozen of us began praying.

About an hour later, my daughter Jeorgi came hobbling in the door, hunched over with a hurt back, too. And then Chris threw out his shoulder and had to go get it popped back in by a chiropractor! They did not have time to work me or Jeorgi in that day, so we were stuck, and I had never received chiropractic care anyway. All we had was prayer. I somehow crawled out of the bed and shouted, "Let the weak say I am strong!" I updated the team and told them to keep praying. I got back into bed and kept typing away about Paul's thorn (chuckling to myself at the damage I must be doing to the kingdom of darkness regarding this subject).

Suddenly, I noticed the wind blowing outside. Then came thunder and a downpour. I turned on the news and sure enough, tornado warnings were issued for my area. Now, I live in a tiny suburb of a big city, and so it is odd to see the name of our little suburb on the news, but there it was, and they were warning us of funnel activity and urging us to take shelter. I texted my children wherever they all were to make sure they were safe.

Everything outside got very still. I have survived five decades of tornado seasons in Nashville and know that this means the worst is about to hit. The calm before the storm. The winds came again, and we watched on the news until the coast was clear. We had no damage, but a friend on the prayer team, Christina, saw the tornado touch down in her neighbor's yard, skip over her house and touch down next door. She was safe. So were we. I then stood up and noticed something amazing. All my back pain was *entirely* gone.

Just like in the back injury story I tell in *Seeing the Voice of God*, I jumped up and down, touched my toes and felt no pain. The last time, God had healed my broken rib and re-inflated my collapsing lung in three days (confirmed by X rays on day five) and this time's back injury only took two. I felt so good I decided to go ahead and do my daily exercises. By the end of the workout I was doing advanced levels. God had done a miracle. I was completely restored!

I am telling you, prayer is powerful and God is the weatherman! Sometimes the two collide. When you war in prayer, it stirs up the heavens. I believe it can even affect the weather. I have seen it again and again in my own life, and you see it in Scripture. An earthquake at Jesus' crucifixion, winds parting waters at the Red Sea, and more.

Maybe you are thinking that you wish God would just do things for you without you having to ask. To which I answer, did you have to ask for salvation? God does not "do salvation" to you, and He is not going to "do healing" to you.

And no matter what, do not beg God for healing. He has already purchased your healing at the cross through Jesus. The Greek word for *salvation* is *sozo* and it means "to save, heal and deliver." So whether you see the word saved or healed in the New Testament, it is most likely this one little word *sozo*. For example: "And besought him greatly, saying, My little daughter lieth at the point of death: I pray thee, come and lay thy hands on her, that she may be healed [*sozo*] and she shall live" (Mark 5:23 KJV); "He that believeth and is baptized shall be saved [*sozo*]" (Mark 16:16 KJV).

So we see that when Jesus gave you the gift of salvation, healing was in the same package. Maybe you did not know it was in there, but now you do! So now you can see that the war on wellness is actually a war on your salvation itself, as well as on the global Gospel. Satan hates the *sozo* package and will try vehemently to steal it from you. Take it back! Stand up and fight! Raise your sword and pray the Word!

We began this section with the Ten Healing Commandments and some of my favorite Scriptures on healing, and now we are ending with a challenge for you to use them to war for your wellness. There is no way around it: Warfare prayer is the "eat your vegetables" of getting healed when resistance is present. It is time to yield and wield.

Corresponding Emotional Toxins

People who constantly have to war for good health deal with ongoing emotions of doubt, weariness, disappointment and frustration. Let's pray now for God to renew your spirit and mind from these potential influences and to help you set new standards for yourself that will benefit your faith:

> *Lord, after reading Your healing Scriptures in this section, there is no doubt that You are my Healer. But the enemy opposes me at every turn, and I am sometimes tempted to doubt that. But I will doubt no more! And I also refuse to be weary, disappointed or frustrated! I will stand up and fight and take back my health today. In Jesus' name, I am healed. Amen!*

Correlating Physical Detox

Today we finish cleansing the lymphatic system. Repeat yesterday's meal plan, experimenting with this section's colors.

Closing Blessing

May God complete the cleansing of your lymphatic system as you win the war on wellness, and just as your lymphatic system helps remove toxins from your body, may the revelation you gain in this section allow you to help rid *the* Body of Christ of its misunderstandings of the healing Gospel.

SECTION **6**

Relationship Toxins

Spiritual Emphasis: Healing the heart from relational grief, while offering practical ideas for reconciliation and family unity that will restore the faith of all involved

Emotions Associated with These Toxins: rejection, neglect, depression, insecurity, anger, discouragement, fear, impatience, humiliation, contempt, guilt, shame, loneliness, embarrassment, grief, despondency, failure

Bodily Systems Detoxed:
Days 19 and 20: Cardiovascular (heart, blood vessels: arteries, capillaries, veins)
Days 21 and 22: Circulatory (blood, all vessels)
Days 23 and 24: Integumentary (skin, hair, nails, sweat glands)

Section Colors

Besides the specified greens, this section's support color is *red*. Red-colored produce is colored by a natural plant pigment called lycopene, which is a bright red carotene and phytochemical found in tomatoes and other red fruits and vegetables. Unlike other vegetables and fruits, where nutrients such as vitamin C are reduced upon processing, cooking tomatoes actually intensifies and heightens the concentration of lycopene.

These hues also contain anthocyanin, which as we studied in Section 5, is a prominent flavonoid that also can contribute blues and purples, depending on the pH level. Anthocyanins are of great value to the food colorant industry because of their ability to contribute vibrant colors to their products. That should come as no surprise considering the vibrancy they contribute to our plates as we consume the health-promoting foods they appear in. You can also eat your way to vibrant skin with the help of these "red," by consuming more apples, beets, strawberries and tomatoes.

Anthocyanins were incorporated into the human diet many centuries ago. North American Indians, Europeans and the Chinese all took advantage of them in their traditional herb treatments, harvesting them from fruits (particularly berries), seeds, roots and dried leaves. They have great antioxidant benefit to the whole body, but have long been known to improve blood circulation, reduce blood pressure, combat heart disease and improve overall cardiovascular health. Is it any wonder with those heart-health benefits that they are red?

Section Grocery List

Purchase one or two of each of the following fruits and vegetables, depending on your appetite level. If the fruit or vegetable is tiny, purchase enough for at least two cups. In the case of leaf vegetables, one head, bunch or bag of each variety mentioned will suffice. You may also double up on one vegetable or fruit if you dislike another, but be open to trying new things! With each section you will better be able to gauge your appetite and adjust your purchases to accommodate it.

Reds	red peppers, beets, radishes, red onion, red potatoes, tomatoes, red apples, cherries, cranberries, red grapes, red grapefruit, raspberries, strawberries, watermelon
Greens	avocado, green pepper, fresh alfalfa, celery, asparagus, endive, spinach, lettuce, turnip, watercress
Allowed Additions	quinoa, brown rice; legumes (red kidney beans, lentils), pineapple, banana, dark chocolate; coffee beans, tossed sparingly into smoothies, if desired; oils: olive, coconut and/or flaxseed; chicken broth; once or twice a week you may trade your veggie snack for a shake (see Recipes)
Herb/ Spice Options	mint leaves (or peppermint oil), garlic, cayenne, ginseng, dong quai, sacred pine, gingko, parsley
Tea	dandelion, milk thistle (see Recipes); booster option: decaf green tea; for flavor add an extra bag of any caffeine-free fruit or berry tea
Optional Meat	only vegetables are recommended, but a three-ounce serving of organic poultry or fish (size of deck of cards) is permitted at dinner
Nuts	walnuts, macadamia nuts, peanuts
Water	drink half your body weight in ounces daily
Bases for Smoothies	choice of milks: organic 2%, unsweetened almond, coconut; choice of waters: coconut or aloe
Rest	nine hours nightly

DAY 19

Spiritual Toxin: B.U.R.D.E.N.E.D. (Betrayed, Unwanted, Rejected, Despised, Evaded, Neglected, Estranged and Discarded)

How is that for a heartbreaking lineup? As I was outlining some thoughts for today's devotional about being forsaken by family or friends, the first few descriptive words from above flowed from my fingertips, and before I knew it I realized they were unintentionally beginning to spell an acronym. "BURDENED." I marveled at what God was saying. I had not thought of giving today's devotional that title, but think of it: What more heartbreaking burden is there than losing a life-defining relationship? The loss is great because the love was great. It truly is like losing a piece of yourself. Let's look at the definition of *burden*: "strain, care, problem, worry, difficulty, trouble, millstone; weigh down, encumber, overload, oppress, harass, upset, distress; haunt, afflict, stress, tax, overwhelm."

Ever experienced any of these burdensome emotions in a relationship? Strain? Worry? Trouble? Oppression? Upset? Stress? Ever felt overwhelmed? Yeah, me, too. I know this may be difficult, but I want you to take a deep breath and go down memory lane with me. I need you to think of a relationship that you have lost in your lifetime. For some of you it was a parent who left, for others it was a spouse who deserted them, and for even more of you it was a friend whom you had invested countless heart hours into and who just turned and walked away. Some of you just pictured three different faces because you have been abandoned multiple times and in multiple ways in life. Rejection leaves behind the initial sting of the desertion, but also the lingering pain of missing the deserter. The pain is as painful as the sweet was sweet.

There is a Bible verse that you hear quoted (in part) quite frequently from Isaiah 53:5 (NKJV): "By His stripes we are healed." I particularly love this verse because one time, the Lord showed me through it that Jesus' blood had such power that it could heal even before Calvary. His stripes alone during the pre-crucifixion beating purchased your health, not to diminish the work of the cross, but to give greater appreciation for the bloodshed of the sacrificial Lamb, Jesus.

But as much as I love this verse, it really is unfair to separate it from the previous two verses, which show *why* Jesus was able to carry this healing anointing. Isaiah 53:3–5 (NKJV):

> He is despised and rejected by men, a Man of sorrows and acquainted with grief. And we hid, as it were, our faces from Him; He was despised, and we did not esteem Him. Surely He has borne our griefs and carried our sorrows; yet we esteemed Him stricken, smitten by God, and afflicted. But He was wounded for our transgressions, He was bruised for our iniquities; the chastisement for our peace was upon Him, and by His stripes we are healed.

Jesus was despised and rejected. He was also betrayed, unwanted, evaded, neglected, estranged and discarded. But when you are thus "burdened," it just means that you are on your cross. Jesus told you to take it up and follow Him, and here you are.

To separate Isaiah 53:5 from verses 3 and 4 (which I do myself all the time) is to separate the guts from the glory. It takes guts to get glory! To disconnect them is to miss the secret behind Jesus' anointing. And if you are not careful, you will miss that your suffering is the secret behind yours, too.

The passage adds that Jesus was a man of sorrow, acquainted with grief, not esteemed, stricken, smitten, afflicted, wounded, bruised and chastised. How on earth did He not call down angels to end the suffering? He chose not to because He knew the anointing was coming. He knew healing was coming. He knew that new life was on its way.

What you must do when you have had a family member or dear friend leave you is to remember that healing and new life are on their way. And a new anointing to love the new companions who will now come alongside, nurture and appreciate you. What you are feeling right now—aside from the pain—is the lack of closure that comes with being discarded. Once when I experienced this, I sat down and wrote this poem as if I were talking to the person(s) that hurt me. Perhaps you might try to do the same thing in your own words. Until then, please use mine:

I wondered if I might, at first
write down my thoughts in rhyme and verse
To find the good this pain has brought
But truth be told, I'm overwrought

I can't pretend a lesson's learned
when all I see are bridges burned
I do not understand God's ways
on this or any other day

He lets me hurt, He bids me pray
but lets you turn and walk away
I hate to say it but it's true:
I need to see Him chasten you

I want fair play, I want it now
I want my day in court, and how
For if it all was read aloud
my case would surely sway the crowd

See, justice is my closest kin
but you need mercy now, my friend
You've set your heart high on a shelf
But in the end, you've hurt yourself

You closed a door and locked it tight
I have knocked and knocked with all my might
I need to turn and walk away
But this last thing I need to say

I would've loved, I would've stood
I would've brought you all things good
I could've served; I could defend
I could've been your perfect friend

I fear for you when no one's left
when you're alone, afraid, bereft
I wonder who'll run to your side
from all those whom you once denied

You'll see your fears were nothing more
than something to be sorry for
And maybe then I'll get to say
the words I am denied today.
© 2007 Laura Harris Smith

Corresponding Emotional Toxins

People who are burdened by betrayals and abandonment often battle rejection, neglect, depression, insecurity and anger. Let's pray now for God to renew your mind and spirit from these potential influences and to help you set new standards for yourself that will benefit your faith:

Lord, my heart loves others in a unique way. It sometimes causes me to expect more than others are willing to give, and it causes me great pain. But today, I am choosing to give You that pain and to forgive. Nobody can be the friend You are to me. Or the parent, spouse or anything. I lay my rejection, neglect, depression, insecurity and anger at Your feet. Bury them at the cross, God. You are my everything. In Jesus' name, Amen.

Correlating Physical Detox

Today and tomorrow we cleanse the cardiovascular system.

Breakfast	The Heart Beet Berry Smoothie
Mid-a.m. Juicing	Laura's One-Two Punch

Lunch	Sixcess Salad
Snack	snack liberally from your reds and greens
Dinner	choose one green and one red fruit or vegetable (see Recipes for prep ideas); pair with brown rice or quinoa tossed with section spices and section nuts or beans
Nightcap	Detox Tea

Closing Blessing

May God cleanse your heart and your entire cardiovascular system as you cleanse your heart from any relationship toxins.

DAY 20

Spiritual Toxin: Unsaved Loved Ones

As Christians, we have the ability to love with a dimension that is so much more fulfilling than ordinary love. If you can think back to how you expressed and felt love before your salvation and then how you express and feel it now, they should be different. Not that you did not love before, but it is as if you went from black and white to color in the intensities of your compassion, vulnerability, loyalty and pleasure. The reason is that you became a new creature. The God who loved the world enough to send His only Son to save it now lives inside of you. It is a beautiful metamorphosis.

But on its heels you quickly begin noticing the non-believers around you and how they do not posses the same aptitude. Oh, they can be kind and charitable and even have beautiful, lifelong relationships, but they cannot comprehend love's fullness until they have died to self and had their *good* love replaced by the eternal *great* love of a heavenly Father.

So when you come to Jesus—or I should say, once you truly allow the love of Jesus to flow fully in your heart no matter how long you have been saved—you become aware of those around you who do not know Him. And because you now have this new love inside you, it creates an internal mourning when you think about not spending eternity with those people you love in this new and extraordinary way. You want them to know Jesus, for this life and for the next. You have a desire to experience the love of God together, and you may even feel a distancing from this person because you cannot. You wonder what you can do.

To that end, I have created a list for you of things you can do to help people have their eyes opened to the love of God and to see them come into full relationship with Him through His Son, Jesus.

1. **First, realize that it is not God's will for this or any other person to perish:** "The Lord is not slack concerning his promise, as some men count slackness; but is longsuffering toward us-ward, not willing that any should perish, but that all should come to repentance" (2 Peter 3:9 KJV).

2. **Remember that in this world of falsehoods and counterfeit spiritual options, God desires all of mankind to know truth:** " . . . who desires all men to be saved and to come to the knowledge of the truth" (1 Timothy 2:4 NASB).

3. **Never forget that your loved one is not resisting you or God but that it is the enemy and his demonic spirits influencing him or her to resist you because of Satan's great contempt for God:** "For we do not wrestle against flesh and blood, but against the rulers, against the authorities, against the cosmic powers over this present darkness, against the spiritual forces of evil in the heavenly places" (Ephesians 6:12).

4. **Pray and inform these spirits that they are not allowed to influence this person anymore:** Scripture says that our binding and losing of these spirits—which is spiritual warfare 101—brings change in the heavenlies, and so since we are fighting "spiritual hosts of wickedness in the heavenly places," through our prayers, remember to pray "binding and loosing prayers" often for them, binding unbelief and loosing faith. "Truly, I say to you, whatever you bind on earth shall be bound in heaven, and whatever you loose on earth shall be loosed in heaven" (Matthew 18:18).

5. **Pray that their eyes would be opened to understand they have a calling, an inheritance and great power:** "I pray that the eyes of your heart may be enlightened in order that you may know the hope to which he has called you, the riches of his glorious inheritance in his holy people, and his incomparably great power for us who believe" (Ephesians 1:18–19 NIV).

6. **Pray that whatever false religion or theology they have studied in the past would no longer blind their minds from the simple Gospel of Jesus Christ:** "The god of this age has blinded the minds of unbelievers, so that they cannot see the light of the gospel that displays the glory of Christ, who is the image of God" (2 Corinthians 4:4 NIV).

7. **Pray for the ungodly friends and bad counsel in their lives to be replaced with godly friends and better counsel:** "Do not let anyone fool you. Bad people can make those who want to live good become bad" (1 Corinthians 15:33 NLV).

8. **Be a good friend and let God's love illuminate your eyes. Remember SALT ("Smile and love them"):** "By this shall

all men know that ye are my disciples, if ye have love one to another" (John 13:35 KJV).

9. **Pray for an open door to share the plan of salvation with them:** ". . . meanwhile praying also for us, that God would open to us a door for the word, to speak the mystery of Christ" (Colossians 4:3 NKJV).

10. **Prepare yourself to share the Gospel with them and to lead them to the Lord:** ". . . always being prepared to make a defense to anyone who asks you for a reason for the hope that is in you; yet do it with gentleness and respect" (1 Peter 3:15). Just tell them it is as easy as "ABC" and ask them if they have ever:

    a. Acknowledged that they need help to live their earthly life and to have eternal life.

    b. Believed that Jesus Christ can give that help and that He is the only way to God.

    c. Confessed that Jesus is Lord of their lives and asked Him into their heart.

If they say no (especially to the last one), tell them forthrightly, "Well, we need to take care of that today. I care too much about you to let you leave here and not know where you will spend eternity and to not know what your full purpose is in this life. This is not about religion but about relationship with God. Can we please pray right now? It is the most important prayer you can ever pray."

If they say yes (I have never had someone tell me no once I put it to them plainly like that), then take their hands and ask them to repeat after you. Tell them they do not have to pray anything they are not comfortable praying (but I have never had anyone stop or back out of anything during it). With your own words or with these below, pray with them repeating after you:

Father God . . . I thank You for sending Jesus into the world. . . . You had a Son but You wanted a family . . . and so You sent Him to get us. . . . I want to be a part of that family. . . . I want You as a Father and I want to spend eternity in heaven. . . . I know that I have not made the best of choices in my life . . . but I ask Your forgiveness and want to start again. . . . Come into my life, Jesus. . . . Take my life and live it through me. . . . I know You are going to make it better than ever. . . . Holy Spirit, fill me now. . . . Be my guide . . . and I invite Your voice into my life. . . . Lead me to the right church where I can grow in You . . . and become a true part of Your family. . . . I am a new creature! In Jesus' name I pray, Amen.

Now, just as there was an "ABC" before you prayed, there is a "DEF" afterward. Tell them they need:

d. Daily time in God's Word (and give them a Bible; yours if you have to).

e. Everyday prayer and time spent listening for God's still, small voice and His promptings.

f. Fellowship with other Christians. Invite them to your church or find them one near their home (this is crucial).

Your unsaved loved ones will not be unsaved for long if you will activate these ten truths and pray for them daily. We will pray together for them in a moment!

Corresponding Emotional Toxins

People who wait for a long time for a loved one to be saved can often experience discouragement, fear and impatience. Let's pray now for God to renew your mind and spirit from these potential influences and to help you set new standards for yourself that will benefit your faith:

Father, I lift up the following unsaved loved ones to You right now. (Just pause and listen to His voice as He brings them to mind. Then, go back to the ten steps and pray each one over each person.) God, I trust You to take all my discouragements, fears and impatience and let those be fuel for daily prayer for these friends and family. In Jesus' name, Amen.

Correlating Physical Detox

Today we finish cleansing the cardiovascular system. Repeat yesterday's meal plan, experimenting with this section's colors.

Closing Blessing

May God complete the detoxification of your cardiovascular system and give you perfect heart health, spirit, mind and body!

DAY 21

Spiritual Toxin: Physical and Verbal Abuse (Unhealthy Environments)

First Corinthians 13:4 (NLV) says, "Love does not give up." Unfortunately, many people abide by this to their own detriment. They love someone so much that they are willing to endure endless abuse and humiliation from them. Verbal and physical (and sometimes sexual abuse). God did not inspire this Scripture with the intent of it causing you harm. Remember that this verse could also apply to you loving yourself and not giving up on yourself, including your well-being and safety.

If you or someone you know is a victim of physical or verbal abuse at home, work or school, today's devotional is intended to bring you (or them) life and hope. If you yourself are the abuser, then it is intended to bring you revelation and conviction enough to make some needed changes in your life. While verbal and physical abuse are not beneficial for anyone, there are some folks who are susceptible to lasting emotional damage if they remain in these environments. Let's start with verbal abuse.

If you have never read *The Five Love Languages* (Northfield, 1995) by Dr. Gary Chapman, it is mandatory reading for you as soon as you finish this book! I mean it! Within it are the five ways that people show and give love, or as Dr. Chapman teaches, "speak and hear love." This book has changed many lives, including mine, and no doubt saved and enriched millions of relationships worldwide. Of the five love languages, there is one called, "Words of Encouragement and Affirmation." These are the people for whom words (each and every one) are of utmost importance. They are heard, tallied and memorized. More important than sweeping the porch for them or giving them a back rub, these folks really just want to be told they are loved, wonderful, awesome and needed, as opposed to being given a gift or asked to "hang out." The good news is, this can come in the convenient form of a quick email, card, phone call or a passing comment in the halls.

I am one of these folks, and "Words of Encouragement and Affirmation" is my love language. It is not that I do not like those other four gestures of love (and the end goal is to become fluent in all love languages), but a "Words" person measures love by the quality and quantity of conversation a person is willing to engage in with them. Not that we want only to be around other talkers (who would do the listening?), but communication plays a key role in our relationships. Arguments are especially unsettling, and we will do anything to drive the conversation to a place of resolution so that closure can be reached and better words remembered. Words can make or break the soul. They can make or break these folks' self-esteem. They can even make or break relationships.

For a "Words" person, verbal abuse is equal to physical abuse. Harmful words leave behind bruises, but worse, because bruises fade but the wounds from words do not. Mark Twain said, "I can live two months on a good compliment." Likewise, an insult can bring two months of mental anguish. Verbal abuse is bad for anyone with any love language, but especially trying for those who need words sewn in to the fabric of their relationships.

Another of the five love languages is "Physical Touch and Closeness." For these folks, one touch, however brief, can define the whole relationship. They are the huggers, touchers (appropriate touching), caressers and lovers of back rubs, foot rubs and of closeness, period. Physical intimacy is also very important within a marriage when husband or wife has this love language.

"Touch" is at the bottom of my list on the love languages' test. It is at the top of my husband's, and "Words" is his last. So we are polar opposites. We joke about having this deal where I scratch his back and he talks to me. Over the years though, I have become a better "cuddler" and he has become a better conversationalist. In fact, he has become a phenomenal public speaker. He can preach circles around me now. I would like to take credit for that, but . . . okay, I will take a little!

For the "Touch" love language folks, just holding hands says, "I love you," in a powerful way. Imagine then, what happens when a person with this love language is the recipient of physical abuse by those same hands. It says, "I hate you." It is emotionally devastating, not to mention physically humiliating and dangerous.

I sometimes wonder if this love language theory is one of the reasons behind why some people stay in physically abusive marriages. True, most of the abused do not know who they are and have serious self-worth issues, but even in that group, some stay and some go. I wonder if the majority of those who do go have the "Touch" love language and cannot survive the devastation from a hit, slap, kick or punch (or worse). Whereas for "Words" me, I might be less emotionally devastated in the long run, not to mention I have the personality that would try to fight back (all threatening 5'2″ of me). But I am telling you, if he verbally belittled or humiliatingly scorned me, especially in public, I would replay the event a million times in my head and have a very hard time forgiving him. Strange, huh? But you see this theory proven true by women who stay with abusive husbands, perhaps because their love language is not "Touch," but "Gift Giving," and so all he has to do is come home with a present and she feels loved again and takes him back.

No matter if you are in a physically abusive marriage or dating relationship or in a verbally abusive one, and no matter what your love language or gender is, you deserve better. The ideal solution in marriage is repentance (from the abuser), restoration (discovering for him or herself why he/she abuses and finding healing) and reconciliation (between husband and wife). But sometimes, you have to go to a safe place while you are being patient for God to work these things out with the individual. I do not believe in divorce, but I have never and will never tell someone to stay in a marriage where his or her life is in danger. Or in a relationship with a parent who physically abuses. Reach out to someone who can take you in or get you legal help. A teacher or pastor is a great place to start. Pressing charges and restraining orders are sometimes unavoidable, too.

If you are in a verbally abusive relationship, why? Proverbs 18:21 tells us that the power of life and death are in the tongue.

Do not stay in friendships or workplace environments where people are constantly speaking death over you, your dreams or your input. And if it is a marriage, pray and ask God for a strategy. Sometimes you can sow seeds of loving words and see change. Other times, you must seek counseling together. I hope you thought more of yourself than to marry someone who degrades you. If not, I speak 1 Corinthians 13:4 over you: Don't give up. On yourself. On them. Seek counsel from a wise Christian friend or counseling from a Christian counselor. *Not* secular counsel who might tell you to give up and cash in your chips. God is a God of justice, but He is also a God of mercy.

If you yourself are a hitter, abuser or degrader, hit your knees. If you are reading this book—a Christian book—you are probably a Christian and are tormented when you find yourself doing these things. Repent to those you have abused. Ask God for help. Seek counseling from a Christian counselor. Begin again. "Know this, my beloved brothers: let every person be quick to hear, slow to speak, slow to anger; for the anger of man does not produce the righteousness of God" (James 1:19–20).

Corresponding Emotional Toxins

People who are in physically, verbally or sexually abusive relationships battle a steady stream of humiliation, fear and contempt. Those who are the abusers wrestle with the residual guilt and shame. Let's pray now for God to renew your spirit and mind from these potential influences and to help you set new standards for yourself that will benefit your faith:

God, I believe it is possible for all of my relationships to be ruled by peace. Mend all of my relationships that need healing from any form of abuse, whether I am the abused or the abuser. I give You any humiliation, fear, contempt,

*guilt or shame I may ever encounter, and I declare that
the Prince of Peace is in our midst. In Jesus' name, Amen.*

Correlating Physical Detox

Today and tomorrow we cleanse the circulatory system.

Breakfast	The Chocolate Cherry Circulation Smoothie
Mid-a.m. Juicing	Four-of-a-Kind Juice
Lunch	Take-Five Stir Fry
Snack	snack liberally from your reds and greens
Dinner	choose one green and one red fruit or vegetable (see Recipes for prep ideas); pair with brown rice or quinoa tossed with section spices and section nuts or beans
Nightcap	Detox Tea

Closing Blessing

May God bless your detox diet and improve the flow of your
circulatory system as you work towards improving the flow of
communication in your relationships.

DAY 22

Spiritual Toxin: The Shadow of Loneliness

Ever sung one of these?

"Sgt. Pepper's Lonely Hearts Club Band" (The Beatles)
"Alone Again (Naturally)" (Gilbert O'Sullivan)
"Are You Lonesome Tonight?" (Elvis Presley)

186

"All By Myself" (Eric Carmen)

"Hey There, Lonely Girl" (Eddie Holman)

"Only the Lonely" (Roy Orbison)

Man, nobody crooned lonely like Roy.

Well, maybe you have not just sung it but lived it. Or maybe you are like me and have a steady stream of people in and out of your house and wish you could be alone sometimes! Maybe you are single, divorced, widowed or even lonely in a home full of people. One thing is for sure, you can feel alone in a crowd. There is a difference between lonely and alone. I would like to speak to each of the four aforementioned groups, one at a time.

Single

It is true that God calls some people to be single. Listen to what He tells Paul in 1 Corinthians 7:32–35.

> I want you to be free from anxieties. The unmarried man is anxious about the things of the Lord, how to please the Lord. But the married man is anxious about worldly things, how to please his wife, and his interests are divided. And the unmarried or betrothed woman is anxious about the things of the Lord, how to be holy in body and spirit. But the married woman is anxious about worldly things, how to please her husband. I say this for your own benefit, not to lay any restraint upon you, but to promote good order and to secure your undivided devotion to the Lord.

But it is also true that He said of Adam: "It is not good that the man should be alone; I will make him a helper fit for him" (Genesis 2:18). (And this verse applies to women, too, because the word here for "man" also means "mankind" in Hebrew.) So which is it? Well, the answer is simple. God wishes that He could have us all to Himself. He wishes we had no distractions.

But He also knows that it is not good for us to be alone. So we are each on a journey with God. Some of us will walk alone with Him. Others will walk with Him while hand in hand with someone else. But for those called to walk alone with God and undistracted, here is the verse He has led me to for you: "For God alone, O my soul, wait in silence, for my hope is from him. He only is my rock and my salvation, my fortress; I shall not be shaken" (Psalm 62:5–6).

Widowed

I have known many people who buried a wife or husband. They have ranged in ages from young twenties to their nineties, and none was easy. Of course, if the spouse knew Jesus, they had hope of reunion. It made all the difference in the world at the funeral.

I would imagine the loneliness after marriage is a different one, for you have tasted the sweetness of marriage and lost it. Now there is no longer a hand to reach for or someone to notice your ups and downs.

Psalm 102:7 says, "I lie awake; I am like a lonely sparrow on the housetop." If that is you, take heart, for God has a promise for you. That very well could include a new spouse, but for now, He is your portion. Here are His words for you today: "Fear not, for I am with you; be not dismayed, for I am your God; I will strengthen you, I will help you, I will uphold you with my righteous right hand" (Isaiah 41:10).

Divorced

So you became one with someone in marriage and gave yourself to that one wholeheartedly. Now that one is gone. If that is a recent wound, you need to know the reason you feel the pain you do is because you have been torn in two. You were "whole-hearted," and now you are "hole-hearted." If it is an old wound, I pray God has healed it. But both groups have felt the sting and indignation of divorce and commiserated with Jesus' words: "Jesus cried out with a loud voice, saying, 'Eli, Eli, lama sabachthani?' that is, 'My God, My God, why have You forsaken me?'" (Matthew 27:46).

As with the widowed and the singles, there may be a spouse for you or God may want you all to Himself from here on out. What is the desire of your heart? Tell God today and remember this promise: "He heals the brokenhearted and binds up their wounds" (Psalm 147:3).

Home Alone

Perhaps you live with a houseful of people and often feel lonely, or with a spouse with whom you are not connecting spiritually, emotionally or physically. Or maybe you are still at home with your parents and feel lonesome and embarrassed as a single still-at-home. Either way, it is a unique form of lonely in which you feel sort of "stuck."

To you full-house-lonelies, I challenge you to say, "When the cares of my heart are many, your consolations cheer my soul" (Psalm 94:19).

To those of you in marriages in which you are waiting for a miraculous revival, God says to you, "For I know the plans I have for you, declares the LORD, plans for welfare and not for evil, to give you a future and a hope" (Jeremiah 29:11).

And to those of you still at home and maybe feeling misunderstood by your parents in your singleness, here is a promise for you: "For my father and my mother have forsaken me, but the LORD will take me in" (Psalm 27:10).

For all of you though, I have been told by my non-married friends that the key is finding people to serve. I urge you to order a copy of *Singled In* (CreateSpace, 2014) by Jeffrey Lee

Brothers, which is a fascinating approach to singlehood in which he claims that singles should not be singled out (as with large singles ministries), but "singled in," spending their time with couples and kids so that they can better learn how to "do family" when it comes their turn (should God will it). Psalm 68:6 (NIV) says, "God sets the lonely in families." So, go get a family!

There are so many more encouragements and Scriptures I need you to hear, but I want you to have them in a more creative way and hear the sound of my voice speaking them to you. So, I want you to watch a video I once created called, "How Did I Wind Up Alone?" It once was on a YouTube channel that was not seen by many, but I am going to bring it out of obscurity and put it on my current Laura Harris Smith YouTube channel just for you to enjoy whenever you would like a friendly voice. View it now at www.youtube.com/watch?v=fbXjvmCo4KQ& index=14&list=PL1KMkGV7DT2liXosFob_7uNUoQNrBGu Cs. Or you can always go to YouTube.com/LauraHarrisSmith and search in The Pin Codes playlist for "How Did I Wind Up Alone?"

As providence would have it, the scheduling of today's devotional has collided with my husband and children all being gone for the day, and I have enjoyed spending this time "alone" with you. I invite you to watch the video and let me encourage you further before the day is out. And remember, get "singled in" and find a family to love on.

Corresponding Emotional Toxins

People who are single, divorced, widowed or still at home often struggle with feelings of loneliness, embarrassment, grief and depression. Let's pray now for God to renew your spirit and mind from these potential influences and to help you set new standards for yourself that will benefit your faith:

Father God, I know You set the lonely in families. Help me to be on the lookout for those people who need me. I surrender any loneliness, embarrassment, grief and depression to You, right now. Help me be on the lookout for others who struggle with these so that I might be a blessing to them. In Jesus' name, Amen.

Correlating Physical Detox

Today we finish cleansing the circulatory system. Repeat yesterday's meal plan, experimenting with this section's colors.

Closing Blessing

May God complete the cleansing of your circulatory system and regulate your blood and circulation as you cleanse and regulate the relationships that He has given you in your life's journey.

DAY 23

Spiritual Toxin: Fatal Faith (Losing Loved Ones)

Have you ever prayed for people to be healed and had them die anyway? It can be fatal to your faith. Perhaps you prayed, fasted, believed, laid hands on them and then they progressively worsened and died. Perhaps they were injured, and you prayed for a miracle that did not come. Why did God allow this? Was it His fault? Was it yours? Was it their fault or some external force, curse or demonic attack they were unprepared for? Long after the casket is closed and the funeral attendees go home, these questions assault your faith.

In fact, they are the enemy's one-two punch. There you are dealing with the death of your loved one and now you are also having to deal with the death of your faith. I have seen it shipwreck the strongest of Christians. I have seen some turn from God because of it. I have seen some rearrange their healing theology because of it. Others silently entertained doubts and after a few more years of accumulated disappointments found themselves unable to believe for the simple things anymore. We have all lost a loved one too soon before. How did you handle it?

Today's topic was the first one of the thirty that God gave me to write when imagining a book about faith toxins. It must be very important to Him for you not to give up on Him when someone dies after you have prayed. It must be very important for you to remember you do not always have all the facts and to trust Him. We must preach the Word of God and not our experience.

Death comes in many different shapes and sizes. The chances are good that you processed your grief and questions in different ways for each loss you suffered. There is death after a long illness, death from a sudden injury, death through abortion, suicide, murder, miscarriage and even the loss of a child you were going to adopt. Each involves a death.

And as if Satan's one-two punch is not enough, there often comes another blow. The triple punch. People approach you and tell you that if you had just had enough faith, your loved one would not have died. Your prayer would have been answered in a different way. They add insult to injury. I have had people say this forthrightly to me while on my healing journey, as if healing never takes time. But it sometimes does. We see in Scripture where Jesus did not always heal people instantaneously with a miracle. In Luke 17, ten lepers asked Jesus to be healed, and He did not do it on the spot. Instead,

He sent them on a journey. While sick! As they were being obedient to Jesus, they were healed. Only one, however, went back to thank Him. This makes me wonder how many of us get sidetracked on our healing journeys. Did the other nine stay well? They never seemed to give glory to God. I wonder.

We do see in Scripture where obedience affects healing. In 2 Kings 5, Elisha told Naaman to dip in the Jordan River seven times and that healing would be his. Once again, God was ordaining a healing journey. But Naaman was insulted and refused. He almost missed his healing. Does this indicate that healing is conditional at times? Perhaps, when God is placing a greater priority on wholeness than healing. But Naaman complied. He humbled himself. He was not healed on the first dip, or the second or the sixth. What was so special about the seventh dip? It was ordained. It was his personalized cure.

So sometimes when we pray and the opposite happens, instead of getting angry with God or deciding never again to believe in the healing Gospel, we need to remind ourselves that we do not always know the full story of people's hearts and lives. Maybe they gave up at the sixth dip. Maybe not even out of pride but out of exhaustion. I have known good, praying people who got tired of their physical battle and truly wanted to go home to God. Days later, they were gone! I wrote the below poem for just such a dear friend, Sheila, upon her death. I pray it ministers to you now.

> It's the age-old question
> We all have asked
> At some point in our praying past
>
> Why are some healed?
> And others, no?
> Why do some stay, while others go?

We're told to pray
We're told to fast
We're told to seek and knock and ask

We build our faith
And learn our lines
And hope for miracles and signs

Then sickness comes
And there you are
Facing illness, injury, a surgeon's scar

But hear me out
And please don't judge
I'd like to give your faith a nudge

The Word can heal
There's power within!
Each denomination has its spin

But when delayed
Or worse, declined
A thousand thoughts race through your mind

Was it his faith?
Was it her sin?
Did she just throw the towel in?

Was it territorial?
Or was it worse?
He forgot a generational curse!

Should I change views?
Should I change pews?
Should I just live my life confused?

Should I lie down?
Should I move on?
Please help me God. My faith is gone.

It's hard, I know
We've all been there
But doubt and faith, the stage won't share

If you lose faith now
If you change your stance
Will healing ever have a chance?

It's best to ask
It's best to believe!
Don't plan to ache. Don't plan to grieve.

Lazarus would say, "Give death a black eye."
Solomon would say, "There's a time to die."

And when you meet Job
He'll be talking to Paul
They'll be talking 'bout timing, and 'bout life's curtain
    call

You'll see all your loved ones
And they'll fill in the gaps
Things you couldn't see here when you had to play taps

There's a time to laugh
There's a time to cry
There's a time to be born and a time to die.

Keep going! Keep praying!
Don't dare give up now!
You made God a promise! He made you a vow!

You're going to live forever!
Though not here, my friend
But you win no matter how life finds its end.

Your faith is too strong for doubt to destroy
So give God your grief
He'll give you his joy

© 2012 Laura Harris Smith

Corresponding Emotional Toxins

People who have lost loved ones under difficult circumstances often wrestle with grief, shock, doubt and anger at God. Let's pray now for God to renew your spirit and mind from these potential influences and to help you set new standards for yourself that will benefit your faith:

Lord, I miss _____. It was hard to lose them, even to You. And it was also hard trying to process the responses of so many people who may have misjudged or misunderstood me and my needs. Right now, I fully entrust You with my grief, shock and doubt surrounding this loss, and I even believe You are strong enough to handle my anger toward You. I am sorry. I am trying. Meet me where I am and keep my faith clean so that I can continue to trust You in the days to come. In Jesus' name, Amen.

Correlating Physical Detox

Today and tomorrow we cleanse the integumentary system.

Breakfast	The Bright Skin Blend
Mid-a.m. Juicing	Warrior Tonic
Lunch	Pick Six Detox Soup
Snack	snack liberally from your reds and greens
Dinner	choose one green and one red fruit or vegetable (see Recipes for prep ideas); pair with brown rice or quinoa tossed with section spices and section nuts or beans
Nightcap	Detox Tea

Closing Blessing

May God bless this cleanse and nourish your hair, nails and skin, as you learn to deal with those people who make you bite your nails, pull out your hair and who are constantly under your skin!

DAY 24

Spiritual Toxin: When Marriage Fails

First comes love, then comes marriage, then comes divorce for half of all those unions. Right? Those are the statistics we have heard for decades, but are they current?

According to NBC's *Today* show, divorce is on the decline in America. Whereas only 65 percent of marriages in the 1970s made it and 70 percent of those in the early '80s, the trend over the last three decades has been that marriage is on the mend. And according to an article they cite from the *New York Times*, the "half of all marriages end in divorce" pop-culture proverb is now a myth. If current trends continue, it will soon be more like one-third. That is right; it appears that almost two-thirds of those taking marriage vows are deciding to keep them.[1]

But wait. What must also be taken into account are the statistics that show that fewer people are getting married to begin with. Many are opting to live together and never walk down the aisle. So are divorce rates (including annulments) really down because marrieds are staying married or because fewer are getting married at all? The number of annual marriages has dropped consistently over time. In 1960, 72 percent of all American adults were married. Today, just 51 percent are. And according to the Pew Research Center, which studies social and demographic trends, "The United States is by no means the only nation where marriage has been losing 'market share' for the past half century. The same trend has taken hold in most other advanced post-industrial societies."[2]

So why are fewer people getting married? A 2010 Pew Research study found that nearly four out of ten Americans felt the institution of marriage was obsolete! True, it is largely due to society's acceptance of other adult living arrangements such as cohabitation, single-parenting and single-person households. But I believe another factor is that people have witnessed the tragedy of divorce and do not want to experience it. The chances are very likely that either a friend, parent, neighbor, church mate, child or extended family member has cried on your shoulder about his or her divorce. If this occurs to you as a single adult, it makes you wonder, "What will happen to me when (and now 'if') I choose to be married?"

Or maybe, divorce has been part of your own life story and you are the one who has cried on shoulders. And whether you yourself have divorced or you are the child of divorce, the devastation has long-lasting generational repercussions. So how does one heal from such devastation?

In all non-mutual divorces, there are the "leavers" and the "lefts." One who wanted the divorce and one who did not. Or sometimes the leaver did not want a divorce but had to flee for safety reasons. But for those individuals for whom marital healing fell out of reach and resulted in divorce, there are multiple emotional passages the heart must navigate through in order to heal and begin again. Here are the reactions you may experience as you heal from divorce. You may feel:

DAZED—You are numb. You fluctuate between questioning if there is something you can do to make the marriage work and mourning the fact that it is unquestionably over. Just as shock victims need first aid after a bomb or earthquake, so do you, body, mind and spirit. Rest and be good to yourself right now.

INCOMPLETE—The loneliness is setting in at this stage and you are feeling like you have lost a part of yourself. Whereas two became one, now that one feels torn in half. It is time for a more intimate relationship with the Lord, and a small group will be of great benefit and support to you, too.

VIOLATED—The practical, everyday inconveniences of divorce are mounting, leaving you angry at the injustices. You did not ask for this financial upheaval. You did not ask for this death to your dream. Now is the time to let faith invade your fury and trust that God will bring you justice.

OSTRACIZED—Certain friends are now awkwardly dodging you because of the details surrounding your divorce. You are mourning the loss of certain friends—even family members—and each one feels like a death. Remember that Jesus was rejected, too (re-read "B.U.R.D.E.N.E.D"). Forgive these people, for they know not what they do.

REGRETFUL—By now you have done some deep soul-searching and revisited everything you wish you had done differently. Learn and grow, but do not stay in this place too long. It is time to forgive yourself.

COMPASSIONATE—In this miraculous phase, you are actually able to look at your ex's past and childhood with new eyes and gain insight into his or her behavior. It evokes pity in you and helps you to not take the behaviors and rejection personally. You finally can forgive.

EXPECTANT—You are in a newfound season of hope. You feel yourself rising from the ashes and putting your life back together. You are a clean page upon which God is about to write "Act II" of your life. Get ready to take the stage and find your spotlight!

Of these healing stages (which spell DIVORCE so you can easily remember them), the first three are about your fears, the next three are about forgiveness and the last one is about your future. That future starts today!

I want to add to this list the importance of prayerfully breaking soul-ties, which we covered in Section 1. Also, know that God has not forsaken you and will not rest until He sees you happy again!

Corresponding Emotional Toxins

People who experience a failed marriage undergo waves of grief, anger, loneliness, despondency and failure. Let's pray now for God to renew your spirit and mind from these potential influences and to help you set new standards for yourself that will benefit your faith:

> *Lord God, divorce is everywhere, it seems. I have had relationships fail and I have tried to comfort others whose relationships have failed. [Pray this if you yourself are divorced:] I give You all the grief, anger, loneliness, despondency and failure that I sometimes feel surrounding my divorce. [Pray this if you are close to someone who has divorced:] I ask that You use me to minister to those who are suffering from the emotions associated with a failed marriage. [And pray this if you are currently married:] God, protect my marriage so that it might become everything You have designed marriage to be. I thank You that You are the lover and healer of my soul and that You will never fail me. In Jesus' name, Amen.*

Correlating Physical Detox

Today we finish cleansing the integumentary system. Repeat yesterday's meal plan, experimenting with this section's colors.

200

Closing Blessing

May God complete the cleansing of your integumentary system and bring results you can see when you look in the mirror, while also bringing you results you can see in the relationships that you hold most dear.

Purpose and Identity Toxins

Spiritual Emphasis: Discovering your God-given identity and discovering what opposes it, seeing yourself from God's balanced perspective and standing tall while proving who you are to your harshest critic: yourself

Emotions Associated with These Toxins: despondency, frustration, impatience, shame, doubt, defeat, pride, bitterness, self-centeredness, disconnection, guilt, selfishness, lust, resignation, ignorance, unbelief, apathy, presumption, indifference, unforgiveness, wickedness, laziness, rebellion, prayerlessness, apathy, detachment, passivity, discouragement, depression, fatigue, rejection, insecurity, anxiety, timidity, fear

Bodily Systems Detoxed:
> Days 25 and 26: Skeletal (bones, bone marrow, joints, teeth, ligaments, cartilage)
> Days 27 and 28: Muscular (muscles)

Days 29 and 30: Sensory (seeing, hearing, touching, smelling, tasting and balance)

Section Colors

Besides the specified greens, this section's support color is *orange*. This color's fresh produce is usually colored by natural plant pigments called carotenoids, which defines a family of about six hundred different plant pigments that function as antioxidants. In autumn, when deciduous trees halt their green chlorophyll production to prepare for winter, their green leaves turn beautiful shades of orange (and sometimes yellow and red) and this is the carotenoids shining through. Plants appear to produce these carotenoids as a means of protection against the sun's harmful rays and energy. Imagine then what they can do to protect your body!

You may not know this, but in the early to mid-1900s there was such a thing as Vitamin P! So where did it go? Now, it is a collective term for a classification of plants known as flavonoids (also called bioflavonoids), which are rich in antioxidants, although they do not operate like conventional hydrogen-donating antioxidants. Their trademark is not staying in the body very long, but just long enough to trigger crucial detoxification enzymes into the liver while also being a toxin magnet to other toxins that "attach" to them and exit the body with them simultaneously. Think of flavonoids like those handy dust mops that attract dirt and get trashed quickly after one use, along with the dust that they collect.

But how do they benefit your sensory, muscular and skeletal systems? Well, of course, you probably heard as a kid that carrots are good for your eyes, and that this is proven by the fact that you never see a rabbit with glasses. It is true! Carrots (and other orange fresh produce) are indeed good for your eyes due to the heavy concentrations of beta carotene, which is a precursor for vitamin A. They are also chock-full of vitamin C, which is yet one more weapon to add to your antioxidant arsenal. Flavonoids are also known to contain anti-spasmolytic agents, which assist in smoothing and relaxing muscles, so we see they are very good for the muscular system. Also, according to a 2012 article published on PubMed.gov entitled, "Flavonoid Intake and Bone Health," a study shows that "flavonoids, found in a wide diversity of plant foods from fruits and vegetables, herbs and spices, essential oils, and beverages, have the most potential of dietary components for promotion of bone health beyond calcium and vitamin D."[1] So, since flavonoids are so abundant in your orange fruits and vegetables, we see that this color is exceptionally beneficial for the skeletal system, as well. Orange you glad?

Section Grocery List

Purchase one or two of each of the following fruits and vegetables, depending on your appetite level. If the fruit or vegetable is tiny, purchase enough for at least two cups. In the case of leaf vegetables, one head, bunch or bag of each variety mentioned will suffice. You may also double up on one vegetable or fruit if you dislike another, but be open to trying new things!

Oranges	oranges, tangelos, papayas, cantaloupes, grapefruit, sweet potatoes, beets, peaches, apricots, orange peppers, carrots, nectarines
Greens	endive, lettuce, spinach, cucumber, celery, green cabbage, avocado, green pepper, fresh alfalfa, asparagus, turnip, broccoli, Brussels sprouts, green peas, zucchini, kale, okra, kiwi
Allowed Additions	quinoa, brown rice; flax seeds, garbanzo beans, butter beans, banana, eggs; oils: olive, coconut and/or flaxseed; chicken broth; once or twice a week you may trade your veggie snack for a shake (see Recipes)

Herb/ Spice Options	cloves, garlic, turmeric, cinnamon, ginger, dill, oregano, cayenne; for hearing loss: gingko biloba, St. John's wort, parsley, vervain, periwinkle, butcher's broom
Tea	dandelion, milk thistle (see Recipes); booster option: decaf green tea; for flavor add an extra bag of any caffeine-free fruit or berry tea
Optional Meat	only vegetables are recommended, but a three-ounce serving of organic poultry or fish (size of deck of cards) is permitted at dinner
Nuts	almonds, walnuts, sunflower seeds
Water	drink half your body weight in ounces daily
Bases for Smoothies	choice of milks: organic 2%, unsweetened almond, coconut; choice of waters: coconut or aloe
Rest	nine hours nightly

DAY 25

Spiritual Toxin: Delayed Deliverance

What exactly is deliverance? Well, it is more than a movie, more than pizza restaurants offer and more than FedEx promises. Still, those provide clues for what true deliverance accomplishes. Like a pizza or a package, you are picked up from one location and delivered to another. Are you addicted to substances? You can be picked up by God and be delivered to a place where you do not crave them anymore. Are you at a job where you are unappreciated and promotion seems to be passing you by? God can pick you up and deliver you to a new job. Are you sick in your body and racked with pain? I am telling you from experience, God can snatch you up and drop you smack-dab in the middle of healing! *That* is deliverance!

Look at this dictionary definition: *Deliverance* means "liberation, release, delivery, discharge, rescue, emancipation, salvation, informal bailout." Did you notice *salvation* in there? That is very telling because in Scripture, the Greek word for *salvation* and *deliverance* are the same, too. As we studied in Section 5, it is the word *sozo* and means "to save, heal and deliver." Such a little word for such a big promise.

It is from the Greek root *sōtēria*, meaning "deliverance, preservation, safety, salvation." So when you see the word *deliverance* in Scripture or *healing* or *salvation* (or their derivatives) it is the same word *sōtēria*. For example: "For he supposed his brethren would have understood how that God by his hand would deliver [*sōtēria*] them: but they understood not" (Acts 7:25 KJV); "Wherefore I pray you to take some meat: for this is for your health [*sōtēria*]: for there shall not an hair fall from the head of any of you" (Acts 27:34 KJV); "That we should be saved [*sōtēria*] from our enemies, and from the hand of all that hate us" (Luke 1:71 KJV).

So do you see that when you received the gift of salvation from Jesus, healing and deliverance were in the same package? Maybe you have never dug down deep enough in the gift bag to know they were in there.

But maybe you *have* dug deep and deeper still and never found your deliverance. In fact, you wonder if Jesus left it out of your gift bag entirely! You have been patient, held on and kept hoping. Maybe you have slipped a few times, but overall, you have never let go of your promise. Remind you of anyone in Scripture?

Moses snapped and told God that He had not kept His end of the bargain when Israel was not being delivered from Pharaoh's grasp. He seemed to forget that when the wills of other people are involved, things take time. Moses had had it. Listen to the anger in his voice:

> Then Moses turned to the LORD and said, "O Lord, why have you done evil to this people? Why did you ever send me? For since I came to Pharaoh to speak in your name, he has done evil to this people, and you have not delivered your people at all."
>
> Exodus 5:22–23

Reminds me of Martha's begrudging words to Jesus when He "failed" to show up in time to deliver brother, Lazarus: "Lord, if you had been here, my brother would not have died" (John 11:21). Soon, Jesus raised Lazarus from the dead. Lots of "wow" at the end of that story, the moral of which is to trust God enough to wait for the "wow." Same with Israel. They were delivered in time to a fertile land, and today that land is a nation. But they did not just arrive to buckets of milk and vats overflowing with honey. It was just pastureland filled with cows and bees! There was work to do. So consider that it is not that your deliverance has not come, but that you are in the stage where God is now requiring you to play your part. It is your job to bring in the harvest. Israel had to bring in their harvest with giants surrounding them in the land. God did not drive them out all at once upon their triumphant entrance into their promised land. Why not? Look at Exodus 23:30 (NIV): "Little by little I will drive them out before you, until you have increased enough to take possession of the land."

And later, He told them the same thing. Look at Judges 3:1–2: "Now these are the nations that the LORD left, to test Israel by them, that is, all in Israel who had not experienced all the wars in Canaan. It was only in order that the generations of the people of Israel might know war, to teach war to those who had not known it before." So, while we know that the enemy is always at work to delay our deliverance, sometimes we see that God is the author of the divine delay because He is teaching us to war.

I wrote this rhyming sonnet recently and pray that it blesses you as you await your deliverance. Remember, I am praying for you.

> Rescue me, oh great God, and set me free
> Liberate my captive heart of its chains
> You are the only One who has its key
> I am the only one who feels its pains

At birth my heart was whole, my spirit too
But one by one the tribulations came
And on their heels came grief before I knew
Then I was left with bitterness and blame
You've saved my spirit; now please save my mind
Erase the fears the years have nursed and fed
Repair the built-in trust that's been maligned
Replace it with salvation in its stead
There are no tactics left to see me through
Deliverance can only come from You

© 2014 Laura Harris Smith

Corresponding Emotional Toxins

People who feel their deliverance is overdue often struggle with feelings of despondency, frustration, impatience and shame. Let's pray now for God to renew your mind and spirit from these potential influences and to help you set new standards for yourself that will benefit your faith:

Father, I know that deliverance comes only through You. You know my situation, Lord. Please lift me up from where I am now and deliver me to a safer, more peaceful place. I give You my despondency, frustration, impatience and shame. I know that deliverance is as much mine as is salvation and healing. Thank You for that! In Jesus' name, Amen.

Correlating Physical Detox

Today and tomorrow we cleanse the skeletal system.

Breakfast	The Bone Fuel Boost
Mid-a.m. Juicing	Laura's One-Two Punch

Lunch	Sixcess Salad
Snack	snack liberally from your oranges and greens
Dinner	choose one green and one orange fruit or vegetable (see Recipes for prep ideas); pair with brown rice or quinoa tossed with section spices and section nuts or beans
Nightcap	Detox Tea

Closing Blessing

May God heal your skeletal system as you learn to stand tall and walk out your deliverance!

DAY 26

Spiritual Toxin: Unanswered Prayers and Unfulfilled Prophecies

Have you ever heard the term *on the up and up*? It seems to have its origins in the late 1800s from sports betting, and according to UsingEnglish.com, the idiom has two meanings:

1. *If you are on the up and up, you are making very good progress in life and doing well.*
2. *To say that something or someone is on the up and up means that the thing or person is legitimate, honest, respectable.*

Well, I created the title to today's topic months ago upon outlining the book, and, in fact, originally it was to be two separate devotionals: "Unanswered Prayers" and "Unfulfilled Prophecies." But as I set forth to write them today, I realized they are the same thing at their core. They both involve waiting and watching. I also noticed that together they form the acronyms *UP* and *UP*. Once I researched that idiom, and based on the idiom's definition, I knew the Holy Spirit was giving me a starting place:

1. *I am to let you know that God wants you to make very good progress in life and do well.*
2. *I am to be totally honest with you about perhaps why your prayers are unanswered and your prophecies are unfulfilled, while giving you legitimate, trustworthy solutions.*

How does that sound? Are you sure you are really ready for #2? I cannot deliver "legitimate, respectable solutions" unless I am honest with you and then you are honest with yourself. I have to stay on the "up and up" with you, and you have to stay on the "up and up" with yourself! Perhaps we should just start first with #2 and look at the hard facts behind why prayers go unanswered and prophecies go unfulfilled.

I said I would be totally honest with you, so here I go: In 2011, I preached a two-part sermon called "Twenty Things That Hinder Answers to Prayer" (http://www.eastgateccf. com/#/im-not/listen). It was—as it sounds—a list of twenty attitudes, practices, doubts or sins that hinder the answering of your prayers and the fulfillment of God's prophetic promises in your life. Few want to address this unpopular issue because of the toes it will step on. But God's Word is full of plenty of "If you . . . then I will" passages. Blessings are often conditional. So I came up with twenty common characteristics I have noticed over the years that people with unanswered prayers seem to have in common. Here are the twenty reasons prayers do not get answered and prophecies do not get fulfilled, and alongside each one, I have now added the name of the evil spirit that I believe influences the attitude, practice, doubt or sin.

Top Twenty Reasons Why Prayers Do Not Get Answered and Prophecies Go Unfulfilled

1. Because of not expecting much to come of them (Doubt).
2. Because of a history of taking credit for something God did (Pride).
3. Because of a secret grudge lodged in the heart against another (Bitterness).
4. Because of not seeking to please the Lord (Self-centeredness).
5. Because of lack of fellowship with God and His Word (Disconnection).
6. Because of unconfessed sin in one's life (Guilt).
7. Because we are not asking within God's will (Selfishness).
8. Because the prayers are designed to fulfill inner lusts, dreams or illusions (Lust).
9. Because of a lack of perseverance (Resignation).
10. Because of a misunderstanding of faith (Ignorance).
11. Because of wavering faith (Unbelief).
12. Because we show no diligence to assist God in the answer (Apathy).
13. Because we presume to know God's timing and prescribe our own solutions (Presumption).
14. Because of uncaring, compassionless attitudes (Indifference).
15. Because of an unforgiving spirit (Unforgiveness).
16. Because of unrighteousness (Wickedness).
17. Because of failure to apply spiritual authority (Laziness).
18. Because of failure to submit to earthly authority (Rebellion).
19. Because of prayerlessness, or not knowing how to pray (Prayerlessness).

20. Because of demonic interference (identify the demonic forces individually by looking for clues at the resistance you are meeting).

If you see any of these playing an active role in your attitudes or practices, deal with the demonic force listed beside it through the prayer of faith. This does not mean that you are demon-possessed, for it is not possible for a Christian who is full of God's Holy Spirit to be possessed by an evil spirit. Satan's influential hosts, however, can whisper, urge and cajole you into one disobedience after another.

And now that I have explained #2 and been "up and up" with you about what might be preventing your prayers from being answered and your prophecies from being fulfilled, I want to remind you of #1: God wants you to make very good progress in life and do well.

You see, God has all the right connections. He can find you the right spouse, solve your financial problems, heal your body, mend your marriage and patch things up with your parents. He can turn your life of war into a life of peace. He wants to answer your prayers, and He wants to fulfill His prophetic words to you! He is your Father in heaven, and you are His child. He loves you unconditionally.

Take solace in the fact that many before you have waited. Waiting on God is an art. Just make sure that God is not waiting on you!

Corresponding Emotional Toxins

People who feel their prayers go unanswered and their prophecies go unfulfilled often wrestle with defeat, along with many of the other twenty forces listed previously. Let's pray now for God to renew your mind and spirit from these potential influences and to help you set new standards for yourself that will benefit your faith:

God, how long will I wait for these prayers to be answered and these prophetic promises to be fulfilled in my life? Reveal to me any place where You are waiting on me! Rid me of the influences of doubt, pride, bitterness, self-centeredness, disfellowship, guilt, selfishness, lust, desertion, ignorance, unbelief, apathy, presumption, indifference, unforgiveness, wickedness, laziness, rebellion and prayerlessness. Replace them with Your Holy Spirit, and answer my prayers in Your perfect timing. In Jesus' name, Amen.

Correlating Physical Detox

Today we finish cleansing the skeletal system. Repeat yesterday's meal plan, experimenting with this section's colors.

Closing Blessing

May God heal your skeletal systems: the bones, marrow, joints, teeth, ligaments, cartilage and all! And may your prayers be answered and prophetic promises fulfilled as you wait patiently on the Lord.

DAY 27

Spiritual Toxin: Ungodly Waiting (God's Contingency Plan)

So far in this section we have talked about waiting on deliverance, answered prayers and unfulfilled prophecies. But there is

214

another kind of waiting. One that wanders aimlessly and does not know for what or on whom it waits. It is not looking for the fulfillment of a particular word or to check another answered prayer off of a prayer list. This person is just waiting for life to find him or her. For identity to appear magically. For purpose to present itself. For destiny to walk through the front door.

You may know people like this. They seem to have no vision. They are all wander and no wonder. It never dawns on them to ask God for anything big. These Christians are waiting for God to do everything for them, including have faith for them, which He will not do. God can inspire you to have faith, but in the end it is your choice as to whether or not you will rise up and claim what is yours. You have a role to play in the process. This is *your* life we are talking about, after all!

Because of the bad fruit I see this type of "waiting" produce in the lives of certain individuals I counsel or pastor, I can say forthrightly that this is an ungodly form of waiting. In fact, it is just plain laziness. God desires to partner with us to bring about everything in the earth. We are all He has to work with down here! If you can fathom the idea, He has designed this world so that He actually needs your help. The entire world hangs upon the free will of man. A risky plan. But one with a very clever outcome, for it calls out the greatness in you when you partner with the greatest Partner on earth and in heaven. Destiny is born.

As if the fact that God partnered with a teenage girl named Mary and put the light of the world in a dark womb is not proof enough that He desires our imperfect partnership, there are other places in Scripture that reveal this, too.

I call these Scriptures, "God's Contingency Plan." They are the "if" passages. Or more specifically, "if you will do this, I will do that" passages. God's part is contingent upon your part. His actions are based conditionally upon yours. While there is such a thing as unconditional love, there is no such thing as unconditional life.

I can give you a dozen instances in Scripture where this took place. Look carefully at these verses and notice all the conditional promises, most of which begin with "if you."

> Therefore, brethren, be even more diligent to make your call and election sure, for if you do these things you will never stumble.
>
> 2 Peter 1:10 NKJV

> "For if you forgive others for their transgressions, your heavenly Father will also forgive you. But if you do not forgive others, then your Father will not forgive your transgressions."
>
> Matthew 6:14–15 NASB

> If my people, who are called by my name, will humble themselves and pray and seek my face and turn from their wicked ways, then I will hear from heaven, and I will forgive their sin and will heal their land.
>
> 2 Chronicles 7:14 NIV

> "I am the vine; you are the branches. If you remain in me and I in you, you will bear much fruit; apart from me you can do nothing."
>
> John 15:5 NIV

> You can pray for anything, and *if you* have faith, *you will* receive it.
>
> Matthew 21:22 NLT, emphasis added

> "*If you* pay attention to these laws and obey them, then the LORD your *God will* continue his covenant of gracious love with you that he promised with an oath to your ancestors."
>
> Deuteronomy 7:12 ISV, emphasis added

"For if you do not believe that I am He, you will die in your sins."

John 8:24 HCSB

The LORD will make you the head, not the tail. If you pay attention to the commands of the LORD. . . .

Deuteronomy 28:13 NIV

All these blessings will come on you and accompany you if you obey the LORD your God.

Deuteronomy 28:2 NIV

In addition, you are saved by this Good News if you hold on to the doctrine I taught you, unless you believed it without thinking it over.

1 Corinthians 15:2 GWT

"If you consent and obey, you will eat the best of the land; but if you refuse and rebel, you will be devoured by the sword."

Isaiah 1:19–20 NASB

"*If you* understand these things, how blessed *you are if you* put them into practice!"

John 13:17 ISV, emphasis added

Friend, do you know what this means? It means that God has put a revolutionary power in *your* hands. *You* have the ability to change your future! We ended "Unanswered Prayers and Unfulfilled Prophecies" with the challenge not to mistake you waiting on God with God waiting on you. But now, let's up the challenge. You have seen that God has a contingency plan in place; now why not create one of your own?

I challenge you to create your own "if You" list and make some vows to God today. "Lord, *if You* give me a better job, *I will* make Your name great there." "God, *if You* give me a child, *I will* dedicate him or her to You." True, we call upon the promises of God and do not need to bargain with God, but what a wonderful way to be just like your heavenly Father. We serve a God of promises. I want to be just like Him. Go ahead. Make your own contingency list. You will find you cannot outgive God.

Corresponding Emotional Toxins

People who are waiting in an ungodly, lazy fashion often feel things like apathy, detachment and passivity. Let's pray now for God to renew your mind and spirit from these potential influences and to help you set new standards for yourself that will benefit your faith:

> *Lord, I do not want to let life pass me by. You have a plan for me, and I want to seize it! As of today, I shake off any apathy, detachment and passivity in Your name, and I ask for You to replace those with a holy drive and passion that can take me where You need me to be. If You will lead me there, Lord, I will follow! In Jesus' name, Amen.*

Correlating Physical Detox

Today and tomorrow we cleanse the muscular system.

Breakfast	The Muscle Flex Protein (Espresso) Smoothie
Mid-a.m. Juicing	Four-of-a-Kind Juice
Lunch	Take-Five Stir Fry
Snack	snack liberally from your oranges and greens
Dinner	choose one green and one orange fruit or vegetable (see Recipes for prep ideas); pair with brown rice or quinoa tossed with section spices and section nuts or beans
Nightcap	Detox Tea

Closing Blessing

May God cleanse your muscular system as you also get moving toward your future, resulting in a stronger you from head to toe!

DAY 28

Spiritual Toxin: Suffering Persecution

Persecution has many forms. Its very definition reveals its multiple faces: *Persecution* means "oppression, victimization, mistreatment, abuse, discrimination, tyranny, harassment, hounding, intimidation, bullying."

The reason I have placed today's devotional in the Purpose and Identity Toxin section is because persecution—that is, discrimination, harassment and bullying related to your Christianity—can erode your self-worth over time and tempt you to change who you are in order to stop the intimidation. Here are a few illustrations, followed by an appropriate verse of comfort.

1. A strained marriage in which one party is persecuted because of professing faith in Jesus and trying to live a righteous life. This person keeps her Christian opinions quiet so as not to stir up division, muffling her voice and the blessing of letting God use it.

> Blessed are those who are persecuted for righteousness' sake, for theirs is the kingdom of heaven.
>
> Matthew 5:10

2. A student who cannot fully express his Christian opinions without being ridiculed or bullied by other students and excluded or denied entrance into certain school

organizations by non-Christian leaders or teachers. He keeps his faith to himself and does not ever fully learn self-expression or evangelism skills.

> "Blessed are you when people hate you and when they exclude you and revile you and spurn your name as evil, on account of the Son of Man!"
>
> Luke 6:22

3. An employee who is restricted from expressing her faith, displaying religious symbols or inviting others to religious events. She may be denied promotions or treated unfairly. She becomes afraid to pray for or minister to other employees around her, and as a result, God is limited from moving in that workplace.

> "For God is pleased with you when you do what you know is right and patiently endure unfair treatment."
>
> 1 Peter 2:19 NLT

4. A righteous politician who is restricted from making decisions based on biblical values without being mocked, rejected and unseated. Change never comes to the region that God promoted him to transform.

> But even if you should suffer for righteousness' sake, you will be blessed. Have no fear of them, nor be troubled.
>
> 1 Peter 3:14

5. A church member who is slandered and shunned for possessing a pure heart and a hunger for more of the Lord by those who resist change and have invited cliquish, political corruption into the church. Revival never comes to that church because only the pure in heart will see God.

> Having a good conscience, so that, when you are slandered, those who revile your good behavior in Christ may be put to shame.
>
> 1 Peter 3:16

6. The recipient of a court verdict on whom an injustice was imposed due to a bias concerning her outspoken Christian reputation. This can result in financial loss, seizure of property, loss of custody or many other distortions of justice.

> Beloved, do not be surprised at the fiery trial when it comes upon you to test you, as though something strange were happening to you. But rejoice insofar as you share Christ's sufferings, that you may also rejoice and be glad when his glory is revealed. If you are insulted for the name of Christ, you are blessed, because the Spirit of glory and of God rests upon you.
>
> 1 Peter 4:12–14

7. Religious oppression and chastisement inflicted upon Christians by government authorities, including interrogation, torture and even martyrdom. Entire countries fail to experience revival when Christians are punished or, worse, killed for their faith in Jesus.

> And the dragon was angry at the woman and declared war against the rest of her children—all who keep God's commandments and maintain their testimony for Jesus.
>
> Revelation 12:17 NLT

8. Spiritual warfare displayed against Christians by Satan in the form of intimidating nightmares, physical illnesses, depression, anxieties, the manifestations of demonic presences in their homes or bedrooms and an overall

persistence to steal peace and wreak havoc in their lives. Many Christians buckle under this spiritual harassment and fail to recognize their authority over Satan's power.

> "Behold, I have given you authority to tread on serpents and scorpions, and over all the power of the enemy, and nothing shall hurt you."
>
> Luke 10:19

During persecution we must remember the words of Ephesians 6:12 (NLT): "For we are not fighting against flesh-and-blood enemies, but against evil rulers and authorities of the unseen world, against mighty powers in this dark world, and against evil spirits in the heavenly places."

In other words, Satan is the author of persecution. Not your boss, your friend, your spouse or your government. Until he is locked away forever at the end of time (see Revelation 20:3), it is the enemy's job description to persecute God's children. "In fact, everyone who wants to live a godly life in Christ Jesus will be persecuted" (2 Timothy 3:12 NIV).

Jesus also warned us that persecution would come by saying things like: "If the world hates you, know that it has hated me before it hated you" (John 15:18); "Love your enemies and pray for those who persecute you" (Matthew 5:44).

In closing, during persecution, never change who you are! Paul's words in 1 Peter 3:15 should be the goal of all: "Sanctify Christ as Lord in your hearts, always being ready to make a defense to everyone who asks you to give an account for the hope that is in you, yet with gentleness and reverence."

Corresponding Emotional Toxins

People who suffer persecution regularly battle ongoing discouragement, depression, fatigue, and rejection. Let's pray now for

God to renew your mind and spirit from these potential influences and to help you set new standards for yourself that will benefit your faith:

> *Heavenly Father, I know You said we would suffer persecution in this life, but I am weary from the constant warring. I have almost grown accustomed to the discouragements, depression, fatigue and rejection, but I am expecting to see a shift as of today. I know that You will never reject me. I know that You are my encouragement and my strength. I also know that I can be confident because You are the glory and the lifter of my head. In Jesus' name, Amen.*

Correlating Physical Detox

Today we finish cleansing the muscular system. Repeat yesterday's meal plan, experimenting with this section's colors.

Closing Blessing

May God finish detoxifying your muscular system as you grow into the person He has created you to be, strong enough to withstand anything. You are an overcomer!

DAY 29

Spiritual Toxin: Copy and Paste (Will the Real Me Please Stand?)

There is so much pressure on this generation. Pressure to perform. Pressure to achieve. Pressure to have the perfect body. Pressure to be the perfect spouse. Pressure to stay young. Pressure to make good grades. Even pressure to be the perfect Christian. All this perfecting can take you miles from the original you and leave you wondering who you really are underneath all the exterior perfections.

If, however, you are hoping that that opener means this is a devotional about slacking off and giving up on becoming the best you, well, you are going to be disappointed. Besides, I think deep down inside you *do* want to be the best you. Why else would you have made it this far in this book?

The difference is all in the perspective. If you are changing and bettering yourself without first confidently knowing who and whose you are, the foundation is unstable and all the changes will not be successful. Nor will you. If, however, you start with the footing of being rooted and grounded in Christ, accepted unconditionally by Him but ever reaching and growing to become more like Him, then your progress and process will be much more fruitful and far less superficial.

I get very frustrated with people who never change or grow. Some of them seem so laid back, easygoing and humble, but the "what you see is what you get" or "this is me; take it or leave it" mindset is the most self-absorbed, narcissistic, vain, self-admiring, egotistical alibi in the world (and yes, all those synonyms were for effect).

So this devotional will not be about never changing due to your love for the original you, but about loving the original you enough to change.

In fact, the "best you" *is* the real you, and that is the person you should be fighting to protect. That person is already within you right now. Michelangelo said, "Every block of stone has a statue inside it and it is the task of the sculptor to discover it." So imagine that the real you is already inside today's you and that God's chisel is merely bringing it definition. With that perspective, from here on out I am going to be addressing *that* you.

Do you even know who that you is? Even if you like the current you, are there ways you can look more like your heavenly Father and be more forgiving? Productive? Loving? Creative? Joyful? Merciful? Disciplined? Sabbath-keeping? I like the current me, but she has a way to go in looking just like her Father. I want to change every single day. I like today's me. I am going to like tomorrow's me even better.

But I remember once when yesteryear's me asked God to please let me be somebody else entirely. Times were hard and I was weary. So hard that food was scarce for the eight of us, and the task of providing it (and the repeated failures) began to make me lose sight of how blessed I already was. Who would not want the blessing of six kids, right? Well, you might say, "Not I!" But if you met my kids, you would want them all. Jessica's strength, Julian's humor, Jhason's steadiness, Jeorgi's loving-kindness, Jude's hair (just kidding; Jude's magnetism) and Jenesis' invincibility. Who would not want a strong, funny, steady, loving, magnetic, invincible household? But all of that was so eclipsed by my struggles that in a pool of tears one day on my knees in my closet, I begged God to let me be somebody else.

What I did not realize was that God *was* turning me into somebody else. The new me was emerging. And once I realized that the new me was the real me, it felt much less like achieving and more like receiving. And of course, I have repented for my tearful wish and thanked God repeatedly for letting me be and keep becoming "me."

I once read that in computing, the phrase *whoami*—which is a concatenation of the words *Who am I?*—is a utility command for a certain operating system. If you have forgotten your username, you merely type in *whoami* to the command prompt window and your identity is revealed, along with your privileges.[2]

Would it not be nice if you could do the same in life? To type in *whoami* and find out who you are? Well guess what? You can!

All you must do is ask God. He will reveal your identity to you, along with all its privileges. You are the only one privileged enough to be you. And you need to know who you are so that when others ask, you know how to answer.

Personally, I like Jesus' mode of operation. He answered questions with questions. ("Who do you say that I am?") In fact, some of His most profound questions came as a reply to someone questioning Him. But He was not asking due to an identity crisis. He knew who He was. He *was* I AM. He still is.

Have you ever been through an identity crisis? According to psychologists, they happen in adolescence. Ever had a midlife crisis? Evidently, those come somewhere from age 37 to mid-fifties. Ever been a victim of identity theft? It is said that more than nine million people each year will!

But with Jesus, you do not have to experience any of these internal crises. He is the giver, definer and protector of your identity. Why? Because He is secure in His. And when you are secure in yours, you can help others find theirs, too. You can help them stay confident when tested. You see, Jesus knew who He was because God affirmed Him. Upon Jesus' baptism, His Father spoke and said, "This is My beloved Son, in whom I am well pleased" (Matthew 3:17 NASB). Jesus left there and went immediately into the desert where Satan tested Him. Satan said, "*If* you are the Son of God, command that these stones become bread" (Matthew 4:3 NASB, emphasis added). Satan wanted to plant doubt in Jesus' mind about His identity. But it did not work. We do not see Jesus saying, "Okay, check out what happens when I zap this boulder." No. Jesus knew that Satan was questioning His identity to get Him to question everything else God had ever said. He did not get caught up in performance to prove who He was. He merely sat there looking like His Father, the great I AM.

If you are going to be a copy-and-paste of anyone, let it be of your heavenly Father. Maybe your earthly father never affirmed you the way God did Jesus at His baptism. Sadly, I hear this repeatedly from broken people all the time. They never heard in their childhoods, "This is my son (or daughter), in whom I am well pleased." In fact, many years ago Chris and I were asked to minister at a large citywide conference on a presbytery prayer team where people lined up to be prayed over. There were three tents designated for this prayer time: one for healing, one for finances and one to receive the Father's blessing. Chris and I were assigned to the last. I remember thinking, *Oh, man! I wish they had put me in the healing tent! That is where all the action and crowd will be.* But to my surprise, the line for the Father's blessing tent was the longest of all three. It wound outside the tent and all the way down the hill. I was shocked. People wept when we merely spoke the love of a father over them.

I speak that blessing over you right now in the name of your heavenly Father—the best father on earth and in heaven—the great I AM. Because of Him, you can know exactly who and whose you are!

Corresponding Emotional Toxins

People who suffer with identity often struggle with feelings of insecurity, anxiety, timidity or fear. Let's pray now for God to renew your mind and spirit from these potential influences and to help you set new standards for yourself that will benefit your faith:

Lord, who do You say that I am? I will not be satisfied with becoming anything less. I give You any insecurities, anxieties, timidity and fear. You know my heart better than I do myself. Make me into the "me" You designed me to be. In Jesus' name, Amen.

Correlating Physical Detox

Today and tomorrow we cleanse the sensory system.

Breakfast	Come to Your Senses Smoothie
Mid-a.m. Juicing	Warrior Tonic
Lunch	Pick Six Detox Soup
Snack	snack liberally from your oranges and greens
Dinner	choose one green and one orange fruit or vegetable (see Recipes for prep ideas); pair with brown rice or quinoa tossed with section spices and section nuts or beans
Nightcap	Detox Tea

Closing Blessing

May God cleanse your sensory system starting with your eyes—physically and spiritually—so that you can see the brand-new you!

DAY 30

Spiritual Toxin: You University

Congratulations! You have reached Day 30 of *The 30-Day Faith Detox*! This book was intended to shake off whatever doubts ailed your faith and spirit, heal your emotions from their residue, and mend your body from its physical manifestations. You have had a whole month to focus on just you, as if you were going back to school at You U! Section 8 will be full of questions about what you have learned so that you can measure your own outcome. It is a no-pressure assessment but is necessary so you can see how far you have come. Plus, we want to determine what you are going to do with all this new and improved faith so that you can begin influencing others with it.

But first, I want to take a look back at what you have done this month. It is quite a lot!

In Section 1, we talked about the force of faith, and you weighed and measured your faith's current condition. I hope you realized that without healthy faith you cannot believe in the miraculous or the supernatural. In fact, without faith, you are not a Christian at all, since it takes faith to become one. In this portion of the book you were reminded that you are made up of three inseparable parts: spirit, mind and body. You also learned that there is a link between what you eat and what you think, between what you think and the condition of your faith, and thereby, there is a very probable food-faith link. It is my prayer that if you were chemically propelling yourself toward doubt through poor food choices, this detox has helped you set better dietary habits and moved you to a majority diet of living foods vs. dead ones.

In Section 2, you set some ambitious goals for the month. How did you do with them? Were you able to give God a tithe of your waking hours and spend an hour and a half working through this book, praying and just listening to Him each day? Did you sleep nine hours each night? It is very likely that you could not do that every night, but at least now it is on your mind to try to make sleep more of a priority. Did you try new vegetables if you were a vegetable hater? And how did you do with those occasional Epsom baths and skin-brushings? Maybe you even bought a portable sauna. The bottom line is that even if you were unable to meet each day's goals, you made *some* changes, and *some* changes lead to even more changes.

In Section 3, you took back control over all of your appetites and unhealthy environments. You examined the media you ingest, which might be infecting your faith. Congratulations if you pruned them from your life. You also learned to avoid ungodly counsel, break soul-ties, keep standing when your heroes fall, avoid church splits and their aftermaths, and I hope you even got a more well-rounded perspective on world catastrophic events and natural disasters. You confronted emotions of doubt, anger, agitation, lust, disillusionment, confusion, uncertainty and fear, and asked God to heal your mind. Finally, you cleansed your digestive, excretory and urinary systems, including your liver. Your bodily filters are now clean! Just imagine what a healthy position that puts you in if you will only maintain it.

In Section 4, you tackled those pesky financial toxins that rob your peace. You learned ten traits of promoted people as evidenced in God's Word. You learned not to sin against God by withholding your tithes from His storehouse, which calls down a curse upon your life and finances. You even learned the ten things *not to do* if you want to stay stuck and never get ahead in life. We prayed a blessing upon your efforts to have and maintain your own home, and you were challenged to have a "stuff liquidation" and redefine "enough." I even shared with you my top twenty Scriptures on what the Bible says about finances so that you can be convinced God is concerned with what you do with them. You faced your fears about money as well as your frustrations, jealousies, anger, rejection, stress, confusion, failures, embarrassments and despairs. In the meantime you cleansed your endocrine, nervous, and reproductive systems as a powerful statement that you are regulating healthier responses to financial strains, increasing your productivity and retraining your brain to embrace the success God has called you to be!

In Section 5, you tackled the health-related toxins with which the enemy has sought to take down you and your faith. You learned the Ten Healing Commandments, which are the cure for sick and tired. Did you memorize them? Never too late! You learned the difference between healings and miracles so that you can understand and not be discouraged when healing takes time. We explored what I believe is false teaching—that Paul's thorn was a disease or affliction God refused to heal him of—and learned how to make your persecution-afflictions work for you and why God allows them to begin with. Then we learned about that little *sozo* word with the big promise of salvation, healing and deliverance, and how the war on wellness is actually a war on your very salvation and on the global Gospel itself. You eradicated the sources of your weariness, disappointments, grief, impatience and anger, while simultaneously detoxing your immune, lymphatic and respiratory systems, signaling to the enemy that you are now more immune to his attacks on your spirit, mind and body.

From Section 6, on relationship toxins, you gleaned the skills to hold your head high and refuse rejection and estrangement with family members and friends. You learned how to pray for your unsaved loved ones and how to respond in unhealthy environments where physical or verbal abuse is present. As a single, single-again, widowed or divorced person, you learned that there is a difference between loneliness and being alone. If from a failed marriage, you gained insight on the seven steps toward finding healing for your heart. And if you lost a loved one too soon in life, you learned to hold on to the healing Gospel and to trust it despite what you saw or see, knowing that God has a plan and is still at work to use the situation for His and your good. You worked through your sorrow, bitterness, rejection, betrayal, loneliness, sadness and more, and since we were discussing the people you love (those in your heart and those who get under your skin), you cleansed your cardiovascular, circulatory and integumentary systems for a fresh start all around.

Finally in this section, Section 7, you asked God about your purpose and identity. You discovered what might be delaying your deliverance, and how to stay on the "up and up" concerning your unanswered prayers and unfulfilled prophecies. You learned how to wait on God, how *not* to wait on God, and how to hold on to Him during the many faces of persecution (which Jesus said would come to us). You even learned about finding your identity in Christ so that no identity thief can steal your purpose for being on this earth. You have tackled your insecurities, frustrations, despondencies, discouragements and embarrassments and taken them down! You are even fresh on the heels of the detoxification of your skeletal, muscular and sensory systems, reminding you to stand tall and see yourself as the "you-nique" person God has created you to be!

As you now move into Section 8, I am going to ask you some inspiring questions, and you can determine how effective you think this detox was for you and where you should go from here. If you feel you did not complete a particular faith-detox offered to you during a devotion, the good news is that you can go back at any time and repeat that day, and I encourage you to do the accompanying bodily detox regimen and pray the prayers for emotion healing, too. In fact, you can isolate any portion of this book at any time for a booster shot in your faith. Are you ready? Let the results begin!

Corresponding Emotional Toxins

People who complete a thirty-day faith-building devotional guide for the spirit, mind and body are filled with hope and resolve! Expectancy and faith! So this time, I am going to pray for *you* so that we can guard what you have accomplished and hear from the Lord on what to do with all this newfound faith. You ready?

Right now, in Jesus' name, I ask God to put a hedge of protection around your spirit, your mind and your body. You have taken the initiative, invested the time and resources into this book, prayed the prayers, prepared the detoxes, and now I am asking God to add His super to your natural and bless your efforts. Father, bless these efforts! You say in Your Word that without faith it is impossible to please You, so, Father, reward this obvious display of obedience with newfound faith! And add to that newfound healing, opportunities, love, promotions, finances, wisdom, wellness, unity and answers. Thank You for the journey, God, and now I entrust my friend to You in this new season. In Jesus' name, Amen!

Correlating Physical Detox

Today we finish cleansing the sensory system. Repeat yesterday's meal plan, experimenting with this section's colors.

Closing Blessing

May God finish the cleansing of your sensory system—your sight, hearing, taste, touch and smell—while increasing your spiritual senses to be able to discern His direction for your new faith-filled walk with Him.

SECTION 8

Day 31

In these thirty days, you have evaluated your faith and the trials that have bombarded it in five main areas of your life: (1) social influences, (2) your finances, (3) your health, (4) your relationships and (5) your identity. Before that, in Sections 1 and 2, you learned some new things about total temple health and how what you eat affects how you think, which then directly affects your faith. You have been challenged, spirit, mind and body!

Now it is a new day. Day 31! It is the first day of your life with a toxin-free faith that is spiritually sound, emotions that are healed from previous pains and a body that is detoxified and has set new habits! You are now a stronger, sharper, more focused child of God. The sky is the limit for you!

With that exciting progress in mind, I want to ask you some thought-provoking questions about your journey. You listened to me for thirty days, and now you need to listen to yourself.

You need to have a frank conversation with the new you about where you are going from here.

The following questions are conversation starters. You can convey the answers in one of three ways:

1. Write them down in a journal.
2. Speak them aloud to God in prayer.
3. Discuss them with a friend, one at a time.

While I can see the benefit of each, I suggest that you include #3, even if you choose #1 or #2. The reason is that it builds accountability so that you might maintain everything you have worked so hard to accomplish this month. Maybe you even went through this thirty-day detox with a friend, as suggested, so that you can continue to process your results together.

The questions are simple. The answers may be simple, too, but do not let your simple answers eclipse the profound outcomes. Are you ready to look at the fruit of the last 720 hours? I am excited for you to see the answers!

I hope you will also share some of your answers with me. Remember to go to my Facebook author page wall (www.Facebook.com/LauraHarrisSmithPage) and let me know what God has done in you these last thirty days—spirit, mind or body. Let the world know! Here we go.

Q&A

Section 1: Look at your old diet and determine the ratio of living foods to dead foods. Review these definitions, if necessary. In the last thirty days, your percentage has been 100 percent living food! So after one month of eating whole foods, can you tell a difference in the way you feel or think? And has your unclouded thinking led to unclouded faith? Explain. And post your thoughts for me!

Section 2: What were your favorite new foods from this month? What is the most significant change you have seen in your body in the last thirty days? Greater energy? Weight loss? Clearer skin? More rested? Better digestion? Greater immunities? A changed palate? List all changes and make note of the new foods that will become part of your weekly grocery list.

Section 3: This important section's faith-detoxing devotionals were not only the first but the longest. Name any changes you have made in your media intake. That includes all television, music via radio or devices, talk radio, magazines, books, news and all forms of social media. Which new changes can you make?

Section 4: What did you learn about your finances this month? About promotion? And what about sharing, gifting or selling your "stuff"? Finally, what did you learn about tithing? Are you a tither? Why or why not?

Section 5: Did you have any health-related breakthroughs this month? Did you learn the cure for "sick and tired"? Do you feel able to give a defense for why Paul's thorn was not a chronic disease or affliction? Finally, see how many of the Ten Healing Commandments you can remember. And memorize the rest so that you will know what to do when sickness comes knocking!

Section 6: Did you experience any new insights about the relationships in your life? About how to handle rejection, abuse or loneliness? Are you praying the Scriptures listed over your unsaved loved ones? Finally, has your faith healed from losing that loved one too soon in life?

Section 7: Do you feel you now have more faith to address your unanswered prayers and unfulfilled prophecies? Do you feel more educated on deliverance and persecution? Finally, what new things did you learn about yourself in this section, and in this last month?

Remember, I want you to post your victories, recipes, breakthroughs and feedback: www.Facebook.com/LauraHarrisSmith Page.

A Well-Deserved Blessing

I want to leave you with a blessing. You have earned it! I am so proud of you for embarking upon this journey, and humbled that you would trust me to accompany you. If I were with you now I would lay my hands on you and pray for a fresh filling of God's Holy Spirit. If you are able, get somewhere quiet and let me pray this final blessing over you.

> *In the name of the Father, Son and Holy Spirit, I speak a newfound energy to your spirit, mind and body. He is three, and so are you, in His image. I declare that what you started here, you will continue, and that Christ will complete the good work begun in you. I declare that your social influences are pure, your finances are plenty, your health is sound, your relationships are whole and your identity is secure in Christ Jesus. You are clean! Your faith is strong! "Now may the God of peace Himself sanctify you completely, and may your whole spirit and soul and body be kept blameless at the coming of our Lord Jesus Christ" (1 Thessalonians 5:23). In Jesus' name, Amen.*

Recipes

Experts' opinions vary greatly on which color vegetables and fruits benefit which organs, but I have arranged and assigned them to the body systems based on my personal research as a starting place for your easy remembering. The good news is, all colors and their nutrients are represented in this book, so you will benefit from every one by the end of it!

Make sure to review the "Yes, Please" and "No, Thanks" lists from Section 2.

BREAKFAST SMOOTHIES

Stevia is my preferred choice for these recipes because it is a natural, zero-calorie sweetener, so use it to bring extra guilt-free sweetness to any dish, especially my smoothies and shakes (or experiment with small amounts of agave, honey, coconut crystals or grade B pure maple syrup).

Yogurt is chock-full of living enzymes, but I generally do not include it in smoothies for two reasons: (1) new studies show that blending disrupts and destroys its living enzymes, and (2) a banana and a milk provide the same consistency and are more flavorful. Substitute with 1 cup yogurt if you prefer, but fold in after blending other ingredients.

Smoothie Base for All Smoothies

½ cup	milk or water (milks: organic 2%, unsweetened almond milk, coconut milk; waters: coconut water, aloe water or filtered water)
1 Tbsp.	olive oil, flaxseed oil or coconut oil (each provides different flavors, so experiment)
½ cup	ice

Note: Blend all smoothies on high until smooth, using additional milk or water if necessary. Consider adding a raw egg for morning protein if you are worried about feeling weak. I don't ever find I need one, but if you do, choose organic. Never store smoothies; drink fresh.

The Yummy Tummy Trimmer Smoothie

	Smoothie Base (choose a milk)
1	banana
½	avocado
½ cup	fresh pineapple
	juice of 1 lemon
¼ tsp.	chopped ginger root
2 Tbsp.	honey
	(for more sweetness, add stevia or agave)

Bottoms Up Detox Smoothie

	Smoothie Base (choose a water)
	handful of spinach
2	yellow apples with peel, sliced
½	a peeled lemon
⅛ tsp.	cayenne pepper
½ tsp.	turmeric

The New Kidney on the Block Blast

	Smoothie Base (choose a water)
2	bananas
2	peeled kiwis
15	cranberries
½	cucumber (with peel)
½	a peeled lemon
¼ tsp.	chopped ginger root
1 Tbsp.	cilantro (or parsley)
½ tsp.	turmeric
1 Tbsp.	honey
1–2 tsp.	powder stevia
	(blend until kiwi seeds disappear)

Endocrine Energy Boost

	Smoothie Base (choose a milk)
2	bananas
30	coffee beans (regular or decaf)
2	raw brown eggs
1 tsp.	powder stevia
4 tsp.	grade B organic maple syrup (or blackstrap molasses)
½ tsp.	cinnamon (optional, but cinnamon boosts the endocrine system)
	(more stevia for sweetness)

Brain Boosting Banana Choco Chip Smoothie

	Smoothie Base (choose a milk)
2	bananas
2 square inches	dark chocolate bar (at least 75% cocoa)
	(optional 20–30 coffee beans, regular or decaf)
2 Tbsp.	honey
	(for more sweetness, add stevia or agave)

The Hormone Fixer Elixir

Smoothie Base (choose a milk)

½ cup   cashews
2   bananas
1   brown egg
1   cup kale
½ tsp.   cinnamon
¼ tsp.   turmeric

Love Your Lungs Smoothie

Smoothie Base (choose a water)

2 cups   purple (or red) grapes
1 cup   pomegranate arils*
3 drops   peppermint flavoring or oil or 3 peppermint leaves

*It is next to impossible to separate the pomegranate seeds from their yummy pulp. These are called "arils." So toss your pomegranate arils in the blender first, blend on high, pour off the liquid and trash the gritty seeds. Then return juice to blender and add other ingredients. This is one of the most uniquely flavored smoothies I have created and I want you to enjoy it.

Lick the Spoon Immune Purple Slurp

Smoothie Base (choose a water)

1 cup   seedless concord grapes (or just purple or red grapes)
1 cup   blueberries
1   cubed plum
1   banana
½ cup   almonds or pistachios, etc.

The Clean Spleen Cider

The spleen loves warm foods. Cold or frozen foods mean more work for this body filter and result in what some call "spleen damp." So to target and nourish the spleen, foods must be cooked or at least brought to room temperature. With that in mind, today and tomorrow's breakfast smoothie is not a smoothie at all, but a cider. I have also placed this spleen detox to fall when you are enjoying your Pick Six Detox Soup for the next two days. Your tonsils and lymph nodes will enjoy the warmth, too!

No Smoothie Base today. Fill blender with:

2 cups	purple (or red) grapes
1 stalk	celery, chunked
½ tsp.	cinnamon
2 tsp.	powder stevia

Warm 2 cups cranberry juice on the stove (not juice cocktail)
Pour over berries in blender
Blend and sip

The Heart Beet Berry Smoothie

	Smoothie Base (choose a water)
2 cups	strawberries
1 cup	red grapes
¼	of a large beet
¼ cup	almonds, pistachios or walnuts
¼ tsp.	cayenne

The Chocolate Cherry Circulation Smoothie

	Smoothie Base (choose a milk)
1 cup	pitted cherries
1 cup	red apple slices
1 cup	strawberries
2 square inches	dark chocolate bar (with at least 75% cocoa)
1 tsp.	powder stevia

The Bright Skin Blend

	Smoothie Base (choose a water; coconut water is great for skin!)
1	avocado
1	banana
1 cup	kale
1 cup	fresh pineapple
4	mint leaves
	juice of 1 lime
1 Tbsp.	honey
½ cup	almonds
½ cup	or more water

The Bone Fuel Boost

	Smoothie Base (choose a milk today for bones; almond milk has about 15 percent more calcium than dairy)
1	orange
½	grapefruit
1 cup	kale
1	banana
1	large romaine lettuce leaf
1	large carrot
1	raw egg
½ cup	almonds
3 heaping Tbsp.	honey

The Muscle Flex Protein (Espresso) Smoothie

	Smoothie Base (choose a milk)
2	bananas
1 Tbsp.	nut butter of choice
1	raw egg
20	coffee beans (or more peanut butter)

Come to Your Senses Smoothie

	Smoothie Base (choose a water)
1	large carrot
1	peach
1	orange
½	avocado
½ cup	spinach
3 tsp.	stevia powder
	add ½ more cup water
	(add any of this section's "hearing herbs" if you suffer from hearing loss or ringing in ears)

JUICINGS

(sweeten with stevia if desired)

Laura's One-Two Punch

Using your section colors, chop 4 cups of one vegetable of your choice, then 4 cups each of 2 fruits of your choice. Juice together and drink immediately, but do not gulp.

Four-of-a-Kind Juice

Using your section colors, juice 4 fruits, add 1 section spice and drink immediately.

Warrior Tonic

Using your section colors, juice 1–2 cups each of all (or a majority) of the green vegetables and add 1 Tbsp. apple cider vinegar (raw and unfiltered). The tonic will not be sweet, but add an apple or two for flavor.

LUNCHES

(If you cannot eat all you have prepared,
stop when full and store the rest for the next
day's lunch, or eat it for a snack later.)

Sixcess Salad

Dice 1 cup each of 6 of your section color's fruits and vegetables and combine with 6 cups of a dark leafy green lettuce of your choice. For dressing, drizzle with olive oil, apple cider vinegar (raw and unfiltered) and fresh citrus juice of choice. Sprinkle with any of your section spices and sea or Himalayan salt.

Take-Five Stir Fry

Choose 2 cups each of 5 vegetables from your section's list. Dice and sauté until tender in skillet with 2 Tbsp. olive oil and ½ cup water. Add sea or Himalayan salt and section spices or herbs to taste, or for international versions, try:

Italian: oregano, basil, garlic, rosemary, thyme, bay leaf
Asian: turmeric, ginger, chilies, wheat-free soy sauce (Tamari brand)
Mexican: cumin, onion powder, cilantro, coriander, chilies

Pick Six Detox Soup

Select 3 cups each of 6 vegetables from your section's list. Place in large pot and fill 3 inches above vegetable line with filtered water or low-sodium chicken broth. Add sea or Himalayan salt, along with your choice of the section's herbs and spices. (Refrigerate second serving for next day.)

DINNER MEAT ENTRÉES

As I have said, during this detox, it would be beneficial to your body to abstain from meat (including fish). Remember that only organic chicken, turkey and fresh fish or fresh frozen fish from healthy sources are allowed.

Meat (Poultry) Entrées

Lean poultry (chicken or turkey) should be baked, sautéed, grilled or broiled. Whichever meat and method you prefer, drizzle with olive oil, add any section spices or herbs and cook with medium heat.

Reed's Nut-Encrusted Fish

Anne Reed, M.S., N.C.

1 lb.	any variety fish cut into 3 oz. fillets
½ cup	nuts, finely ground (pecans, almonds, walnuts . . .)
3	egg whites
	spices (Herbamare or section's spices)

Rinse and pat very dry. Rub in spices of choice. Dip fish in egg whites then roll firmly in nut meal, baking at 275° for 20–30 minutes. Fish is done when it flakes easily with fork.

EXTRAS

Godfather's Healing Soup

Dr. Rucele Consigny

In a slow cooker, lay a 3–4 lb. whole chicken on a bed of:

1	sliced onion
4	celery pieces, halved
2	carrots, halved
3	whole garlic cloves

Add 1 cup chicken broth.
Dribble desired olive oil over chicken.
Sprinkle with Worcestershire sauce.
Dust with salt and fresh-ground pepper.

Slow cook on low 8–9 hours. Remove chicken, saving broth and ingredients. Peel off meat and return bones and unwanted chicken pieces to broth. Add 2 cups water or broth and bring to boil. Simmer covered for 4 to 5 hours. Strain with colander and discard solids. Strain again with fine sieve or strainer. Add to the clean broth:

4	carrots, sliced thickly
2	potatoes, diced
½	onion, diced
2 Tbsp.	fresh parsley
1 tsp.	red pepper flakes
1 Tbsp.	dried chives
	pulled chicken, to taste

Bring to boil and simmer for 13 minutes or until carrots are tender. Salt and pepper to taste. This is a very chunky, hearty soup. Feel free to add more water or organic chicken broth to dilute.

Tam's To-Your-Health Roasted Vegetables (use for any veggie combo)

Tamara Rowe, The Wellness Coach

Drizzle 2 lbs. of beets, Brussels sprouts, onions, etc. (small pieces/wedges of any vegetable) with 1 Tbsp. extra-virgin olive oil. Sprinkle with sea salt/pepper to taste. Place in 425° oven for 40–45 minutes. Use for any veggie combo!

Sautéed Vegetables

See "Take-Five Stir Fry" for ideas on stovetop preparation of vegetables.

Fruitful Salad

Janice Harris

1 cup	orange sections
1 cup	pineapple cubes
1 cup	seedless green grapes, halved
½ cup	blueberries
1 cup	unsweetened shredded coconut

Dressing (whisk together):

2 tsp.	lemon juice

1 tsp.	grated orange rind
2 Tbsp.	honey
1 cup	yogurt

Stir into fruit and refrigerate for at least an hour.

Then add:

½ cup	sliced strawberries
1	banana
	toasted almonds

Quinoa and Brown Rice

As a delicious side dish for evening meals, prepare 1 cup of brown rice or quinoa per package instructions and in final 7 minutes of cooking add pine nuts, chopped garlic and section herbs or spices. Quinoa is preferred because it is a complete protein, meaning it provides all nine essential amino acids necessary for good health. Gluten-free, its nickname is "the mother grain."

Cashew Rice and Peas

Dr. Jim Sharps, N.D., H.D., Dr.N.Sc., Ph.D.

brown rice
curry powder
roasted, salted whole cashews or cashew pieces
cooked peas

Cook the brown rice using the package directions or the rice cooker directions, but use canned vegetable broth instead of water and use olive oil instead of plain oil. Add curry powder to the rice water before you cook the rice. When the rice is done cooking, stir in the cashews and cooked peas and serve.

Orange Jasmine Rice

Dr. Elisa Ramirez-Sharps, N.D., C.C.H., C.N.C.

2 cups	jasmine or brown rice
1 14-oz. can	vegetable broth
½ cup	orange juice

½ cup	water
2 Tbsp.	sesame oil
1 tsp.	powdered ginger
¼ tsp.	sea salt
¼ tsp.	onion powder
¼ tsp.	garlic powder

Put the rice in a fine sieve and run water over it until the water coming out of the strainer is clear, not cloudy. Allow the rice to drain for a minute. Put all ingredients in a rice cooker and cook until the rice is plump and tender.

SNACK SHAKES

All shakes are blended until desired consistency using additional milk or water if necessary.

Shake Base

½ cup	organic milk or almond milk
1 Tbsp.	honey
½ tsp.	powder stevia (more to taste)

Baby Banana Split Shake

	Shake Base
1	banana
6	strawberries
½ cup	pineapple (optional)
¼ cup	nuts of choice
1 tsp.	unsweetened cocoa powder
1–2	fresh cherries on top

The Carrot Cake Shake

	Shake Base
2	carrots, chunked
1 tsp.	cinnamon

½ tsp.	nutmeg and cloves
1 tsp.	vanilla extract
2 Tbsp.	walnuts

If your carrots are large, add more milk so that the shake is not too thick to slurp up through a straw.

Peanut Butter Jelly Time Shake

Shake Base

½ cup	no-sugar-added grape juice
4	strawberries
2 Tbsp.	creamy peanut butter (or PB2 powdered peanut butter)

Good Mornin' Sunshine Shake

Shake Base

½ cup	papaya
2	large oranges
	(add ½ cup cantaloupe for a tropical flavor)

DRINKS

Nanny's Fruit Punch

Janice Harris

2 cups	unsweetened apple juice
2 cups	unsweetened pineapple juice
1 cup	fresh orange juice
¼ cup	lemon juice
	lemon slice and mint to garnish

Trish's Cleansing Potassium Broth

Trish Beverstein

To remove toxins from the body, alkalinize and re-mineralize the system.

3	jalapeños, deseeded
4 bulbs	garlic, peeled
2	large onions
4 stalks	celery
5 lbs.	carrots
1 bunch	kale
3	beets, with greens
3 lbs.	potatoes, with skins

Bring a large pot of filtered water to boil. As water heats, fill with **chopped** veggies, including favorite spices and sea salt. Water should cover veggies.

Cover and simmer gently for 1 hour. Remove from heat; leave lid on pot. Let sit for another hour.

Strain and sip on liquid all day, as desired.

Fountain of Youth Detox Water

(Counts toward your daily water quota.)

1	cucumber, thinly sliced
1	lemon, sliced
1	orange, sliced
10	mint leaves

Add to 1 pitcher filtered water and let sit overnight.

Nightcap Detox Tea

Brew 1 tea bag each of dandelion root and milk thistle in 1–2 cups water and add 1 Tbsp. honey or stevia. Sip before bedtime. Add a bag from any tea recommendations on your section's grocery list, or sip them during the day.

Dandelion is known in Persia as "the little postman" because it always brings the body good news, gently cleansing it whenever sipped. Traditional Medicinals makes a healthy Roasted Dandelion Root Tea.

Milk thistle's main ingredient is silymarin and is both an anti-inflammatory and antioxidant. Alvita makes a hearty milk thistle tea.

Celestial Seasonings makes a Natural Detox Wellness Tea containing both dandelion and milk thistle, plus echinacea, red clover, roasted barley, licorice, roasted chicory and sarsaparilla.

Notes

Section 1: Faith and Physics

1. "Why You Should Detox With Whole Foods," *The Dr. Oz Show,* October 21, 2014, http://www.doctoroz.com/episode/plan-detox-without-juicing.

2. Harvard Medical School, "The Gut-Brain Connection," *HealthBeat*, accessed July 14, 2015, http://www.health.harvard.edu/healthbeat/the-gut-brain-connection.

Section 2: Prepare to Be Amazed

1. "Microwave Oven Radiation," U.S. Food and Drug Administration, last modified October 8, 2014, http://www.fda.gov/Radiation-EmittingProducts/Resources forYouRadiationEmittingProducts/ucm252762.htm.

2. Our meter measures microwave radiation from .01 mW/cm^2 up through 1 mW/cm^2. TriField, the maker of the meter we purchased, says that studies suggest biological effects may begin to occur near .1 mW/cm^2 of microwave power (TriField Meter Model 100XE instruction manual, page 3), so .5–1 mW/cm^2 is too great a threshold to gamble with.

3. University College London, "New Evidence Linking Fruit and Vegetable Consumption with Lower Mortality," ScienceDaily, March 31, 2014, http://www .sciencedaily.com/releases/2014/03/140331194030.htm.

4. Kathleen Doheny, "The Truth about Fat," WebMD, July 13, 2009, http:// www.webmd.com/diet/the-truth-about-fat?page=3.

Section 3: Social Influence Toxins

1. Kidney Treatment, "Is Mango Good for Chronic Kidney Disease Patients," January 18, 2014, http://www.kidney-treatment.org/ckd-diet/521.html.

2. Anup Shah, "World Military Spending," *Global Issues*, June 30, 2013, http://www.globalissues.org/print/article/75.

Section 4: Financial Toxins

1. "Housing Vacancies and Homeownership, First Quarter," The United States Census Bureau, 2015, http://www.census.gov/housing/hvs/.
2. Marsha L. Richins, "When Wanting Is Better Than Having," *Journal of Consumer Research*, June 2013, quoted in Derek Thompson, "Why Wanting Expensive Things Makes Us So Much Happier Than Buying Them," *The Atlantic*, June 11, 2013, http://www.theatlantic.com/business/archive/2013/06/why-wanting-expensive-things-makes-us-so-much-happier-than-buying-them/276717/.
3. "Scripture on Giving, Etc.," National Christian Foundation, accessed July 14, 2015, https://indiana.nationalchristian.com/816.

Section 5: Health-Related Toxins

1. D. Landsborough, "St. Paul and Temporal Lobe Epilepsy," *Journal of Neurology, Neurosurgery, and Psychiatry*, no. 50 (1987): 662, http://www.ncbi.nlm.nih.gov/pmc/articles/PMC1032067/pdf/jnnpsyc00553-0001.pdf.

Section 6: Relationship Toxins

1. Meghan Holohan, "Divorce Rates Are Lower, but So Are the Number of People Getting Married," *Today Show*, December 3, 2014, http://www.today.com/health/divorce-rates-are-lower-so-are-marriage-rates-1D80332291.
2. D'Vera Cohn et al., "Barely Half of U.S. Adults Are Married—A Record Low," Pew Research Center, December 14, 2011, http://www.pewsocialtrends.org/2011/12/14/barely-half-of-u-s-adults-are-married-a-record-low/.

Section 7: Purpose and Identity Toxins

1. C. M. Weaver et al., "Flavonoid Intake and Bone Health," abstract, *Journal of Nutrition in Gerontology and Geriatrics* no. 31 (2012), http://www.ncbi.nlm.nih.gov/pubmed/22888840.
2. "WHOAMI Utility in Windows 7 and Its Use," The Windows Club, February 11, 2012, http://www.thewindowsclub.com/whoami-windows.

"Faith is the currency of heaven," says **Laura Harris Smith.** "It is the only way to purchase change for your life. Thus, the way to keep from having a boring one is to stuff your pockets full of faith and spend as much as you can as often as you can."

The Chosen author is the founding co-pastor of Eastgate Creative Christian Fellowship in Nashville, Tennessee, along with her husband, Chris.

"Without faith," she says, "we are not even Christians, which is why Satan opposes faith so adamantly and won't relent until he steals it all. So at the core of all my writings are truths that bolster faith and intimate communication with Jesus, with a strong argument for how our salvation should be clearly identifiable by others in our spirits, minds and bodies. If God truly saves us, He saves all three parts. If I am truly His, it illuminates my whole being, not just one-third or two-thirds of me."

Laura is the author of a number of books, including *Seeing the Voice of God: What God Is Telling You through Dreams and Visions* (Chosen, 2014), which stayed at #1 on the Amazon bestseller list for multiple weeks in multiple categories in multiple countries. She speaks and ministers across denominational lines, and is known for bringing a lighthearted look at the heaviest of biblical topics.

Married for 32 years, Chris and Laura have six children, Jessica, Julian, Jhason, Jeorgi, Jude and Jenesis, all home-schooled, walking with the Lord and creative in their own rights. With half of them now grown and married, the "grandmuffins" now outnumber the kids.

Invite Laura to speak: booking@LauraHarrisSmith.com

Official website: LauraHarrisSmith.com
Facebook: Facebook.com/LauraHarrisSmithPage
Twitter: @LauraHSmith
YouTube: YouTube.com/LauraHarrisSmith
Chris and Laura's Nashville Church: EastgateCCF.com

Ready to take the free 30-Day Faith Detox Challenge? Want access to the 30 videos where Laura encourages you daily on your faith detox right from her own kitchen? Make your smoothies, soups, entrées and more with Laura and get prayed for daily during your 30-day faith detox. Just visit:

www.LauraHarrisSmith.com/faithdetox.html

On Day 1 of your detox (once you have completed Sections 1 and 2 and done your grocery shopping), you will be ready to begin the actual faith detox and begin Section 3. On that day (Day 1), go to the above site and sign up for the section emails, and you will automatically receive an email from Laura at the start of each new section during your detox. This is a free, secret link for book purchasers just like you and is Laura's way of saying thanks.

Take the 30-Day Faith Detox Challenge. Take your *whole church or group* through the free 30-Day Faith Detox Challenge! It's a reset button for your body, mind and spirit. Also visit www.Facebook.com/LauraHarrisSmithPage for more details.